DANCE!
Roots, Ritual and Romance

Carmelle Bégin

Pierre Crépeau

CANADIAN MUSEUM   MUSÉE CANADIEN
OF CIVILIZATION   DES CIVILISATIONS

© 1989 Canadian Museum of Civilization

Canadian Cataloguing in Publication Data

Bégin, Carmelle

Dance: roots, rituals and romance

ISBN 0-660-10791-0
Issued also in French under title: Danseries.

1. Folk dancing – Canada. 2. Immigrants – Canada – Songs and music. 3. Dancing – Canada. I. Crépeau, Pierre, 1927-   . II. Canadian Museum of Civilization. III. Title. IV. Title: Roots, ritual and romance.

GV1625.B53 1989   793.3'1971   C89-097083-1

ISBN 0-660-10791-0
DSS catalogue no. NM98-3/58-1989E
Printed and bound in Canada

Published by the Canadian Museum of Civilization
100 Laurier Street
P.O. Box 3100, Station B
Hull, Quebec
J8X 4H2

Édition française
Danseries: portrait de notre culture
ISBN 0-660-90288-5
Publié par le Musée canadien des civilisations

Table of Contents

Introduction	5
PRAYER Ritual Dances	6
Spirit Dances	6
Fertility Dances	11
Healing Dances	14
DRAMA Theatrical Dances	
Dances of India	17
SEDUCTION Dances of Love	21
Tarantella	21
Portuguese Dances	23
Baladi	24
Flamenco	26
IDENTITY Dances of Allegiance	28
The People of the Salons	28
Strings That Bind	30
Dances of Resistance	36
ESCAPISM Dances of Entertainment	40
CONCLUSION Pure Pleasure	47
Descriptions of Artifacts and Photos	48

Photography
    Optima Photographie Enr.: pages 9, 12, 15, 19, 22, 23, 25, 29, 32, 33, 36, 37, 42, 44, 45.
    Richard Garner: cover, pages 7, 10, 11, 16, 26, 30, 31, 34, 35, 39.
    Carmelle Bégin: pages 13, 20, 24, 41 (left), 43, 46.
    J.-P. Camus: page 8.
    J. Lenczewski: pages 18, 27, 38.
    A. Gallaugher and P. Haslebacher: page 41 (right).

Coordination: Nicole Saint-Jean

Editing: Robert P. Allen

Production: Henri Rivard

Design: France Lafond

Printing: Boulanger Inc.

Introduction

Dance is a primal medium of expression. Perhaps the first method of human communication to develop, it is a form capable of expressing, through its combination of rhythms, gestures and colours, the entire spectrum of human feelings and experience: seduction, prayer, joy, grief, worry, threat, imagination, fascination, fantasy, enchantment, ecstasy, fidelity and escape. Every civilization has developed its own dance forms; every era has witnessed the birth of new rhythms and new dance figures; and every sociey has imbued its dances with a national character. Successive waves of immigrants have brought, and continue to bring, the dances and musical traditions of other lands to Canada. As a result, a large number of the world's choreographic traditions are now represented in this country. As they encounter a new physical, social and cultural environment, these traditions and dances undergo change. The functions of a dance, and sometimes its figures and rhythms, will change when moved to a different country. The same is true of the ideas and feelings that dance attempts to express. Simultaneously, these migrations exert an influence on the choreographic panorama in Canada.

This publication presents various musical and dance traditions brought to Canada by immigrants and the changes undergone in the process of adaptation to a new social and cultural environment. In turn, the book shows how these new traditions became contributors to Canada's own artistic vitality.

It is also an opportunity to showcase treasures of the Canadian Museum of Civilization by displaying some of the most beautiful artifacts in its collections. Within the Museum, the Canadian Centre for Folk Culture Studies has an outstanding collection of varied and colourful costumes and its collection of musical instruments is one of the largest of its kind in Canada.

Readers of this text will discover the great richness and complexity of popular dance, the many functions it serves and the infinite variety of its forms. The range of emotions experienced will evoke pride in being part of a nation with such a richly varied cultural heritage.

CHAPTER 1

PRAYER

Ritual Dances

Dance has always been associated with divinity. It was through dance that humanity first attempted to establish relationships with the gods, long before the use of either prayer or song. In dance, the whole body is used to express polarities of experience: hope and fear, rebellion and submission, pain and joy, need and thanksgiving. Fertility dances express both heartrending appeals to Mother Earth and celebrations of her generosity. In spirit dances, there is both ritual intoxication and protective evocation while healing dances evoke curative conjurations.

All these are primal expressions of both identity and communication. By reaching out to the gods, humankind finds its own place within the cosmos and the ritualism so basic to dance expression becomes a means of vital self-identity. This quality is not left behind when a group of people choose to immigrate. They carry with them the inner cosmic identity represented by their rituals but, in the process of integration and relocation, those needs change. In a country like Canada, for example, the ritualistic functions of the dance traditions brought with them by immigrants begin to diminish in importance. But there is still a need for a familiar touchstone — for a way to maintain contact with elements that affirm inner identity. That is why the dance traditions themselves survive. We see them in the forms and figures danced, in the costumes and masks worn by the dancers and in the musical instruments used to accompany the dances. While its primal ritualism may have become much more secular, dance remains the surest and most direct route to contact with a deeper identity.

Spirit Dances

Since the dawn of time, people have tried to establish contact with the spirit world. The best results have always come from rhythm, music, song and, above all, dance. The African hunter's dances of incantation, the joyous village feasts in honour of ancestors and the protracted entreaties of Haitian voodoo are all expressions of the unquenched desire for physical encounters with the spirits.

Cameroonian Drum

Primitive hunters performed a dance to honour the spirit of the animal they were about to pursue. Largely dependent on hunting for their survival, they sought union with the animal world in order to ensure its continuing bounty. This Cameroonian drum is adorned with raised scenes that recall hunting expeditions undoubtedly graced with particular benevolence from the spirits of the ancestors.

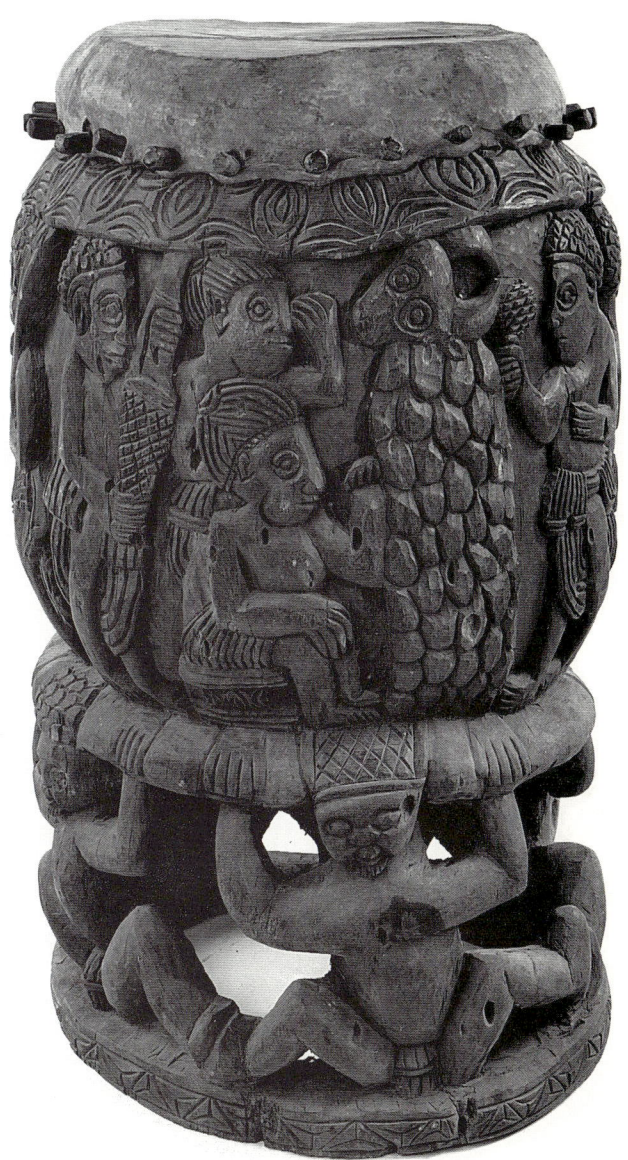

Congo Dancer

Voodoo is a religion of dance. Through dance, Haitians praise their gods and offer them their prayers, entreaties and thanks. They express these various religious sentiments in three great voodoo rituals — *rada*, *petro* and *congo* — each characterized by specific rhythms and varied and complex dance figures. Divine benevolence shows itself by the spirit taking possession of a worshipper who then goes into a trance and is said to be ridden like a horse by the *loa*. Dressed in an *arc-en-ciel* (rainbow) costume recalling the "freed slave" class, this dancer moves to the beat of the *congo*, a rite of love marked by tenderness and elegance.

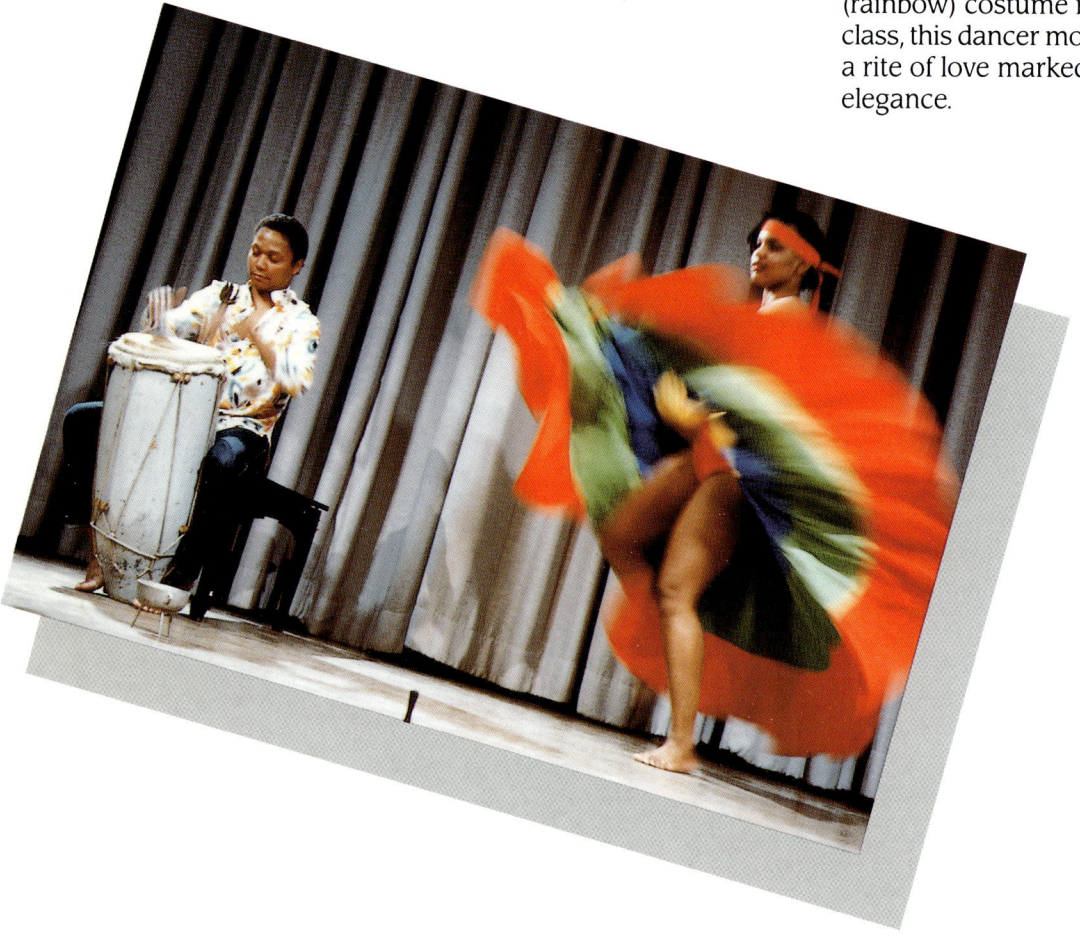

The Haitian Drum

The Haitian drum — the essential voodoo instrument — is sacred, the incarnation of a deity. It is consecrated in a solemn baptism and libations and sacrifices are offered to it. This drum, made in 1954, was imported from Haiti in 1981 by the drummer for the Mapou Ginen troupe of Montréal. Voodoo is practised in Montréal's Haitian community. Although the rituals are performed secretly, some of the dances are performed publicly as affirmations of Haitian cultural identity.

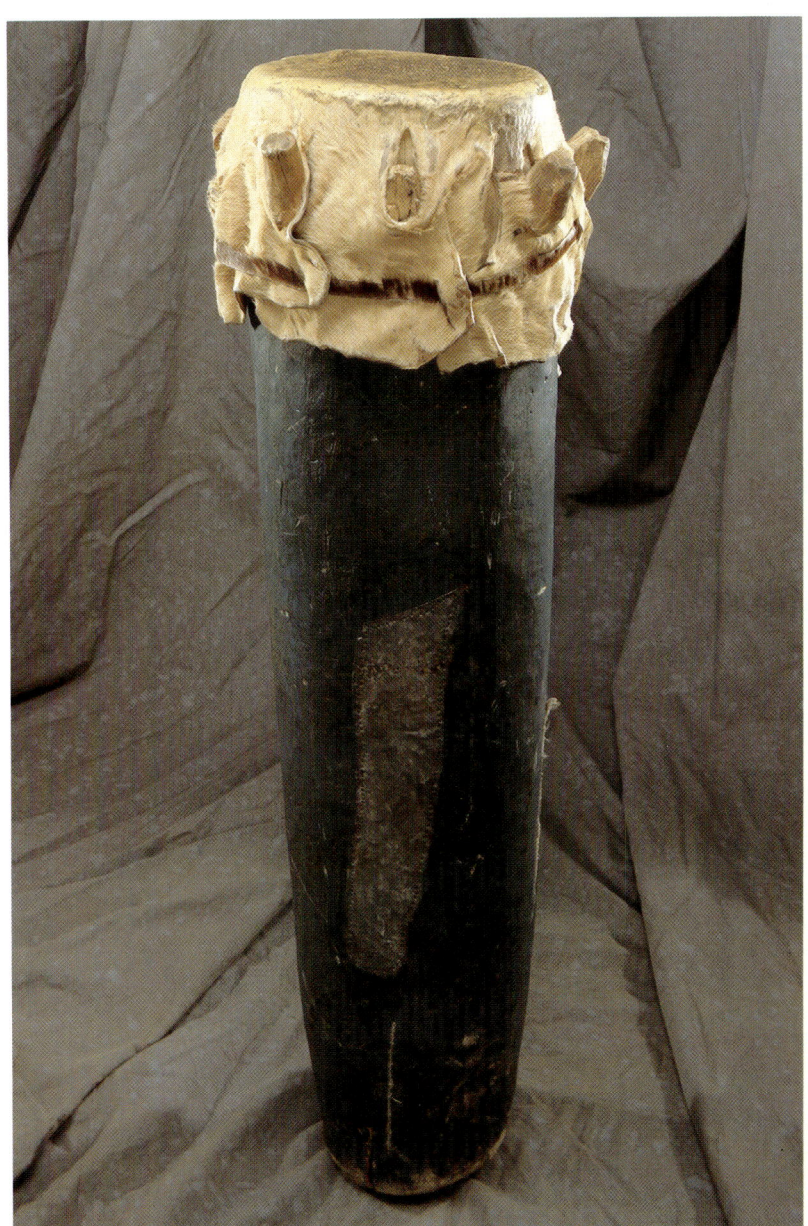

Mmwo Mask and Kalangu Drum

The dances using masks in honour of ancestors sought the benevolent protection of the ancestors' spirits. To wear a mask representing an ancestor is to be possessed by that ancestor's spirit and to bring him or her to life once again in the body of another. The masked dancer becomes the ancestor, alive again within the family. With its delicate features, spectral white face and distinctive hairstyle, this particularly expressive mask of a young woman's spirit bears an astonishing resemblance to some Asiatic masks. A product of the *Mmwo* secret society, this mask is used in ritual yam dances and at funerals.

Use of the *kalangu* drum is associated with specific community rituals. To its rhythms, bodies of the deceased are escorted to their final resting place. At weddings and name-giving ceremonies, young girls dance to the beat of the *kalangu*. It also is the accompaniment for rituals sacred to the butchering of livestock. Community agricultural work is performed with the beat of the *kalangu* providing a rhythmic backdrop. These sacred dances generally are not done outside the native village except in performances shorn of religious significance and intended solely to demonstrate the ethnocultural identity of the dancers. In today's industrialized societies, the mask has lost its value as an instrument of personification and is often nothing more than an ornament.

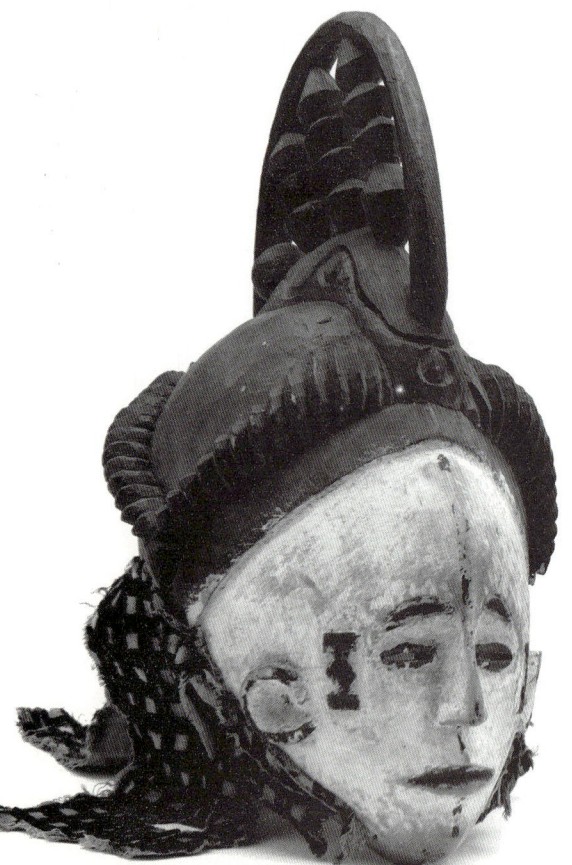
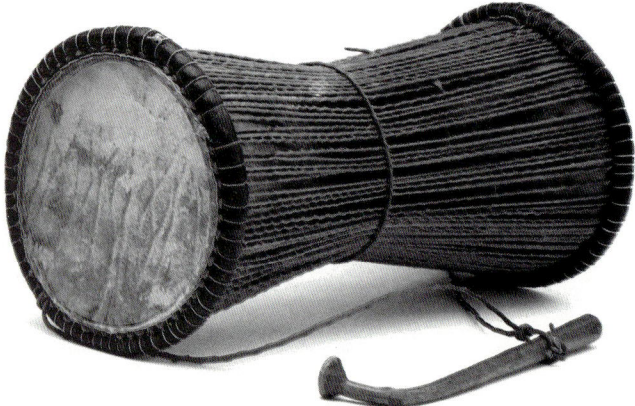

Fertility Dances

Very early in the history of humanity, dance served as a prayer to the gods, an entreaty to ensure the fertility of the soil, herds and people. It was also through dance that farmers expressed their joy and thanked the gods for harvests.

Mask of Nimba

This majestic mask represents Nimba, the great goddess of fertility among the Baga of Guinea. The jutting head, hooked nose and ample breasts are distinctive symbols of fertility. During the ritual dances of the rice harvest, the mask is mounted on the shoulders of the initiate who also wears a wide raffia skirt. The combined effect is a source of irresistible fascination for all the participants.

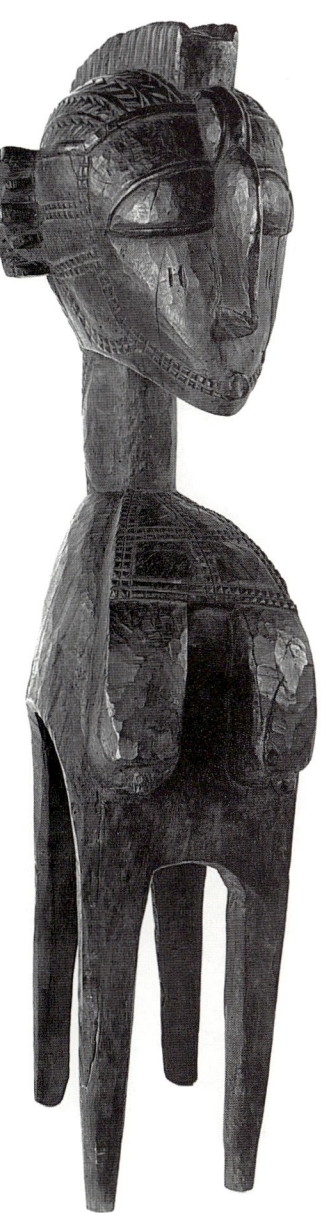

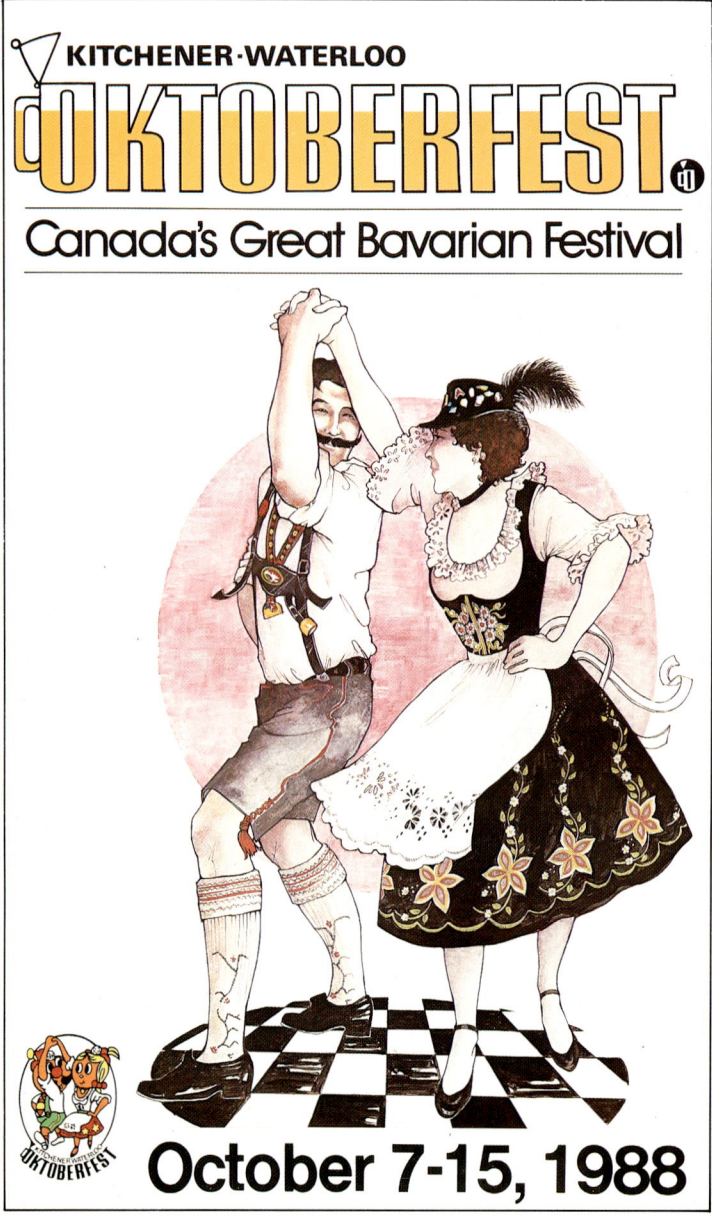

Oktoberfest

Four thousand years ago in Crete, people sang and danced in the centre square of the palace of Minos to thank the deities for the annual harvest. This ancient tradition continued in Europe and, over the ages, was transformed into various regional celebrations such as Oktoberfest and grape harvest and wine festivals. Both have been transplanted to Canada. St. Catharines, Ontario, located in the heartland of Canada's largest grape-growing and wine-making region, hosts its annual Grape and Wine Festival. It runs for approximately ten days at the end of September and dance is an essential element.

Oktoberfest, the Germanic version of these festivities, is related to beer making and the harvesting of hops and grain. In Canada, this tradition is strongest in Kitchener, Ontario, where the Austrian and Bavarian costumes — the *dirndl* for women and the *lederhosen* for men — can be seen everywhere.

Morris Dancers

Every year at daybreak on the first of May, a group gathers in Toronto's High Park to celebrate the arrival of spring and the fertility of the soil through morris dances. Morris dances are part of the age-old tradition of fertility dances. In medieval times, they were unquestionably the most popular dances in rural England but were never allowed at court, probably because of their ritual connotations.

The songs heard during modern performances clearly evoke the original function of celebrating the springtime awakening of nature. In Canada, morris dances also have social and cultural functions; they attest to the permanence of a distinct ethnocultural group. They sometimes are accompanied by the English concertina, accordion, or fiddle, as well as by the flute and drum.

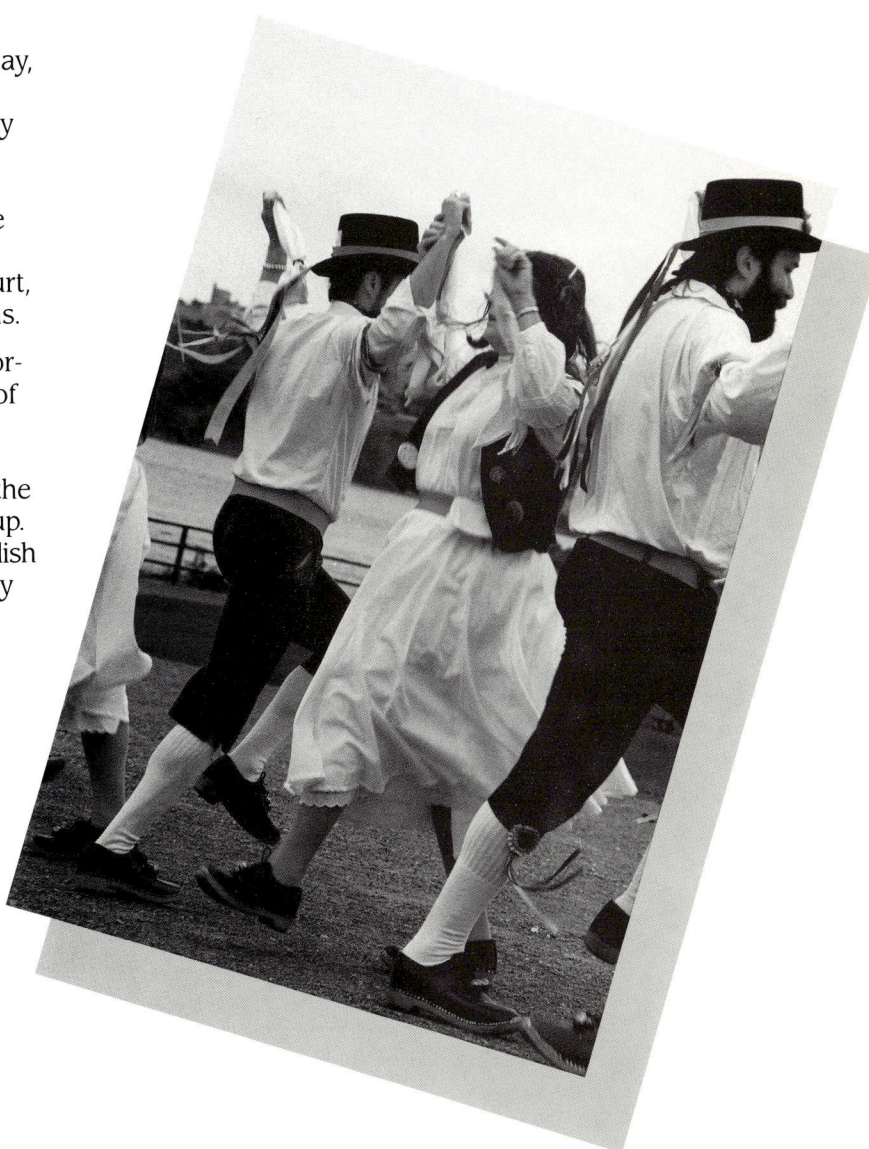

Healing Dances

It is a common belief that possession by a malevolent spirit causes mental and physical illness and that this spirit may be rendered harmless by incantations, the beating of drums and masked dances. The masked dance is not simply the dramatic representation of imaginary beings, either benevolent or malevolent. It embodies the visions, dreams, hopes and fears of a people battling with forces of nature they can neither understand nor master. By neutralizing the mythical power of malevolent demons, the masked dance serves not only as an expression of, but also as an instrument in this constant struggle against the invisible forces that threaten the very existence of the social group.

Cholera Demon Mask and Garula Mask

Sri Lanka possesses an astonishing tradition of masked dance with a range capable of expressing everything from appeasement rituals to the gods to forms of social criticism. There are two main styles of masks — the *sanni* and the *kolam*. The *sanni* is a mask with contorted human features representing the various symptoms of illnesses while the *kolam* represents mythical characters, animals and supernatural beings. Recent masks generally display innovations but continue to be inspired by familiar images of tradition. In Canada, the masks convey the same references to traditional mythology but are adapted to a different social and cultural environment. These two *kolam* masks are among the most spectacular of all Sinhalese masks.

The first is the mask of the great cholera demon, Maka-Kola-Sanni-Yaka, god of all spirits, master of all illnesses and cause of a wide range of afflictions. It is entreated primarily when an illness cannot be diagnosed. The eighteen masks which encircle the central mask represent the demons of the major illnesses. This mask creates a spectre of terror for the viewer.

The second, the Garula mask (eagle mask), is decorated with geometric designs and feathers. Garula is the Sri Lankan version of the Indian Garuda, a mythical bird human in form with an eagle's beak, that served as the god Vishnu's mount. It is worshipped as a destroyer of snakes.

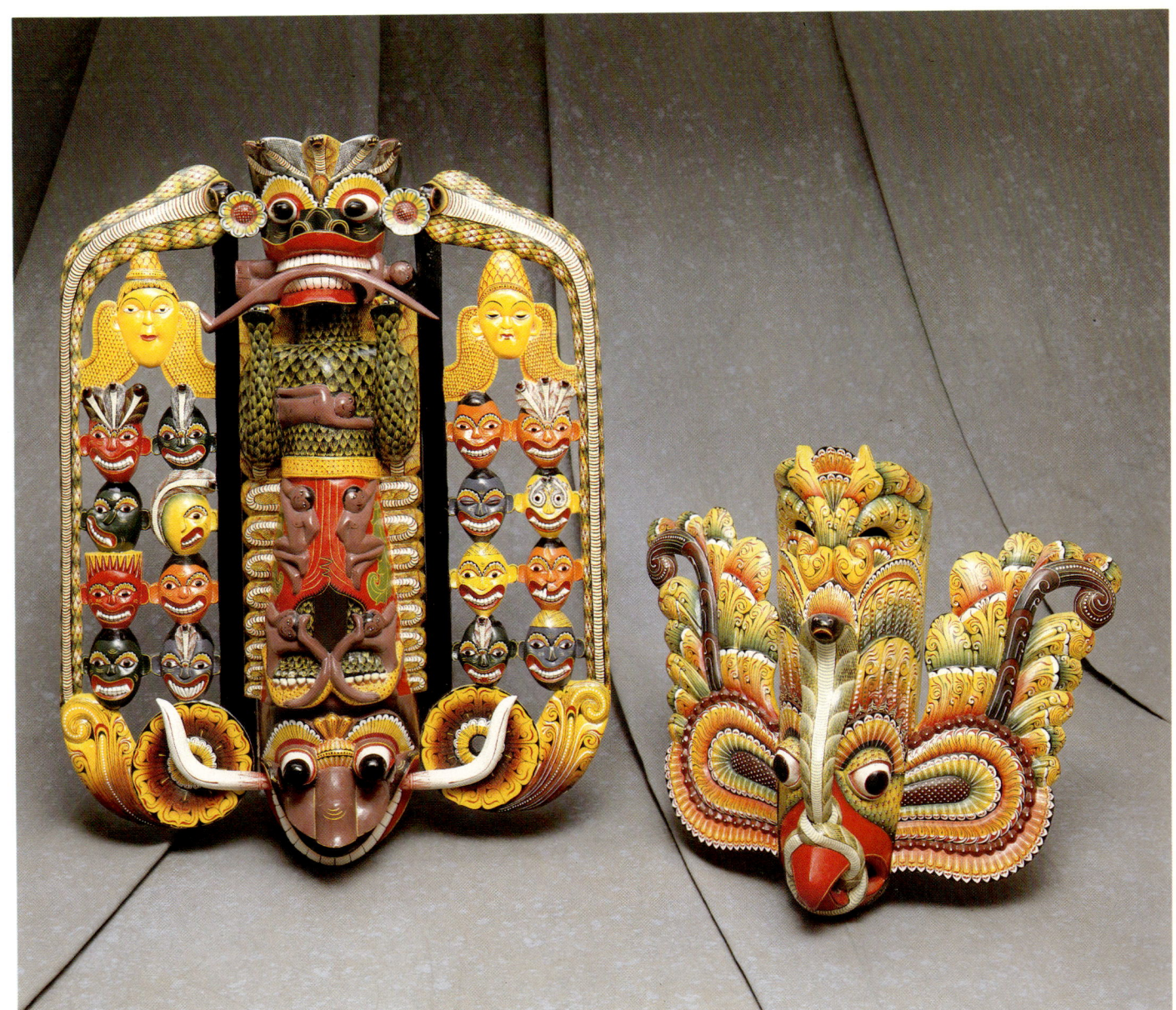

15

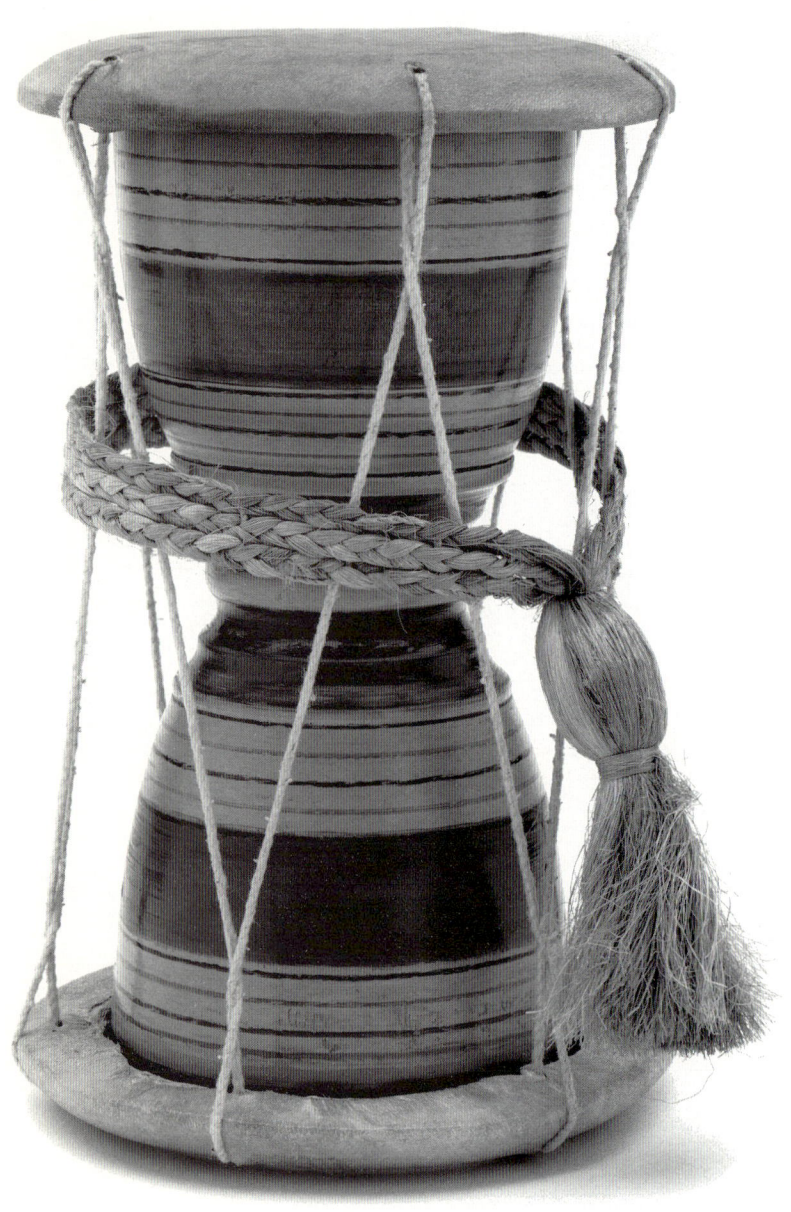

Udakki Drum

Until recent times, the Sri Lankan masked dances associated with healing rituals were accompanied by the *udakki* drum. Today, the *udakki* is used primarily in the region of Kandy, Sri Lanka's religious centre, where it accompanies a typical dance called the *udakki* dance. The dancer simultaneously sings and plays the drum with the dance movements echoing the beat created on the drum.

CHAPTER 2

DRAMA
Theatrical Dances

The cultural heritage of every civilization includes a collection of myths and legends which serve mainly to justify human actions and the current state of affairs. Such dances represent more than mere memory and recollection of creation myths, legends, local stories and feats performed by national heroes. The intent is to revive and resurrect the actual experiences. That strong narrative and mystical generality is evident in such oriental dances as the Bharata Natyam of India, a dance descended from age-old traditions.

Dances of India

Some of the oldest and most remarkable choreographic traditions in the world come from India and the subtlety, complexity and virtuosity of Indian dance is matched by its antiquity. Bharata Natyam — an integration of rhythm, movement, language and emotion — is perhaps the oldest of India's classical dances. Shiva himself is said to have revealed it to the world almost 8,000 years ago and, until the mid-nineteenth century, the great temples and princely courts of India maintained dance troupes which gave impressive performances depicting traditional myths and legends. Today, Bharata Natyam is usually a solo dance accompanied by special music in which voice plays an essential role. In telling a story or recounting an event, the singer provides the dancer with subjects for improvisation. The dancer then describes an element of the narration — place, character or feelings — with her gestures and poses. She personifies the heroes of the forest, the plants, the ferocious beasts, fear in the face of the unknown or daring in the face of danger. The singer is accompanied by the *vina* lute or by a group of instruments including the bamboo flute, the *mridanga* drum and the small *tala* cymbals. Bharata Natyam, with all its splendour, sophistication of rhythms and finesse of figures is now well established in Canada.

Daisy Sahoo Performing Her Arangetram

The first solo performance of a young Indian dancing girl is called an *arangetram* and, as part of an age-old sacred tradition, represents a rite of passage. Because of its grace and beauty, Bharata Natyam has attracted acclaim and admiration from all Canadians who have seen it performed in this country. Here is Daisy Sahoo in a classic pose during her initiation in Ottawa on October 17, 1987. Daisy studied under guru Vasanthi Srinivasan, founder and director of the Natyanjali school in Ottawa.

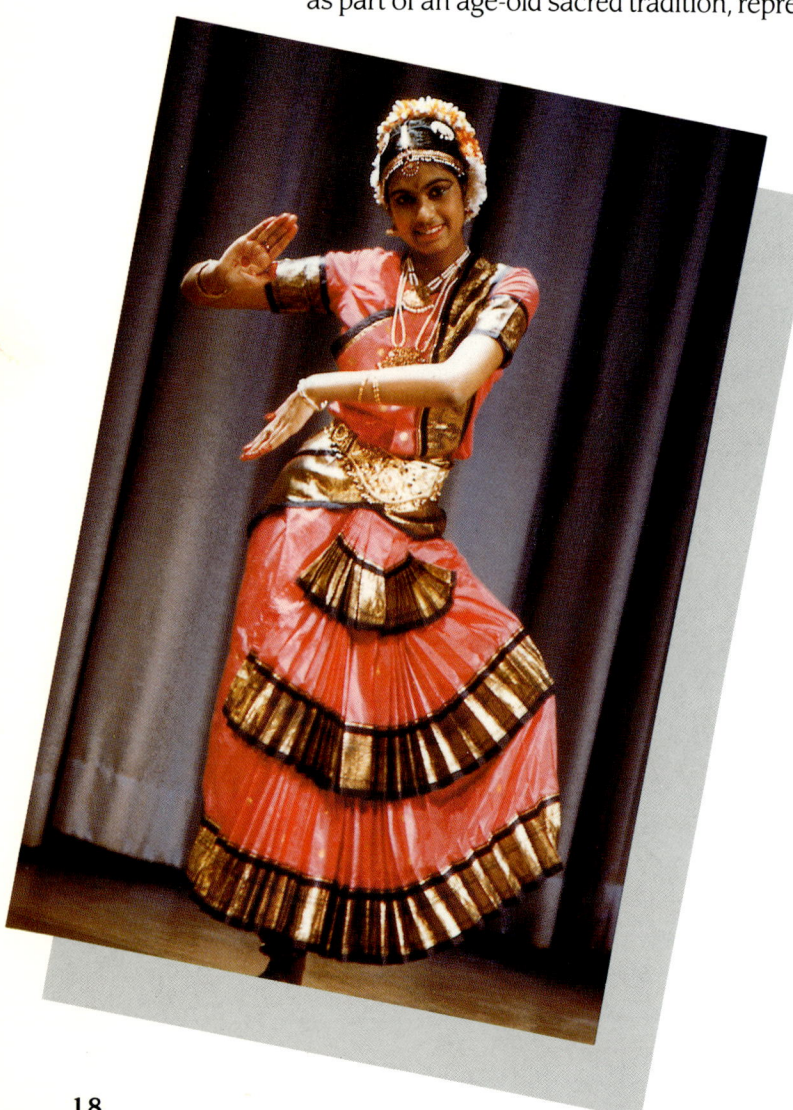

Vina Lute and Mridanga Drum

Vina Sarasvati, the name given to this long-necked lute, refers to the icon of the goddess Sarasvati in the act of playing this instrument. This icon, displayed in most music schools in southern India, signifies that the learning of music leads to an understanding of life's essence and permits the individual's liberation from the cycle of reincarnation. This type of *vina*, called a Tanjore vina, is characterized by its light-coloured wood, carved designs, the head of the dragon-like Yali at the end of the neck and the bright colours of the gourd that serves as the resonator.

The *mridanga* is the classical drum of India. It accompanies songs and the movements and gestures of actors and dancers, using rhythmic patterns of infinite tonal range, colour and detail and structured much like a language. The drummer, sitting cross-legged with the *mridanga* resting horizontally in front of him, also may give a solo recital with pieces lasting fifteen minutes to an hour without ever repeating the same rhythmic pattern.

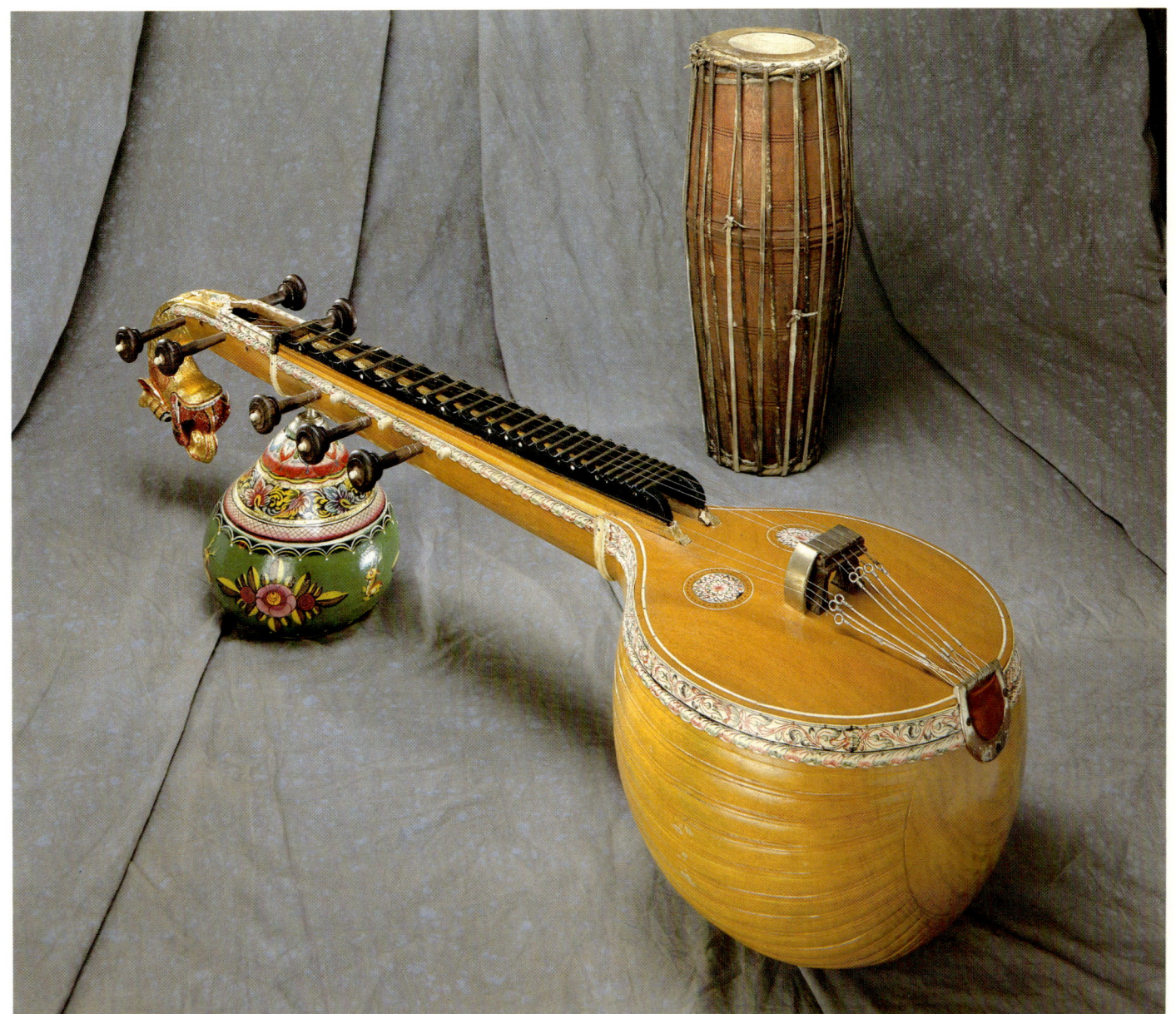

Mudra

The skilful movements of the dancer's hands are symbolic gestures called *mudra*. They illustrate the myths and legends that form the narrative of the Bharata Natyam. There are some four thousand different *mudra* described in the Natya Shastra, the two thousand year-old Indian dance manual.

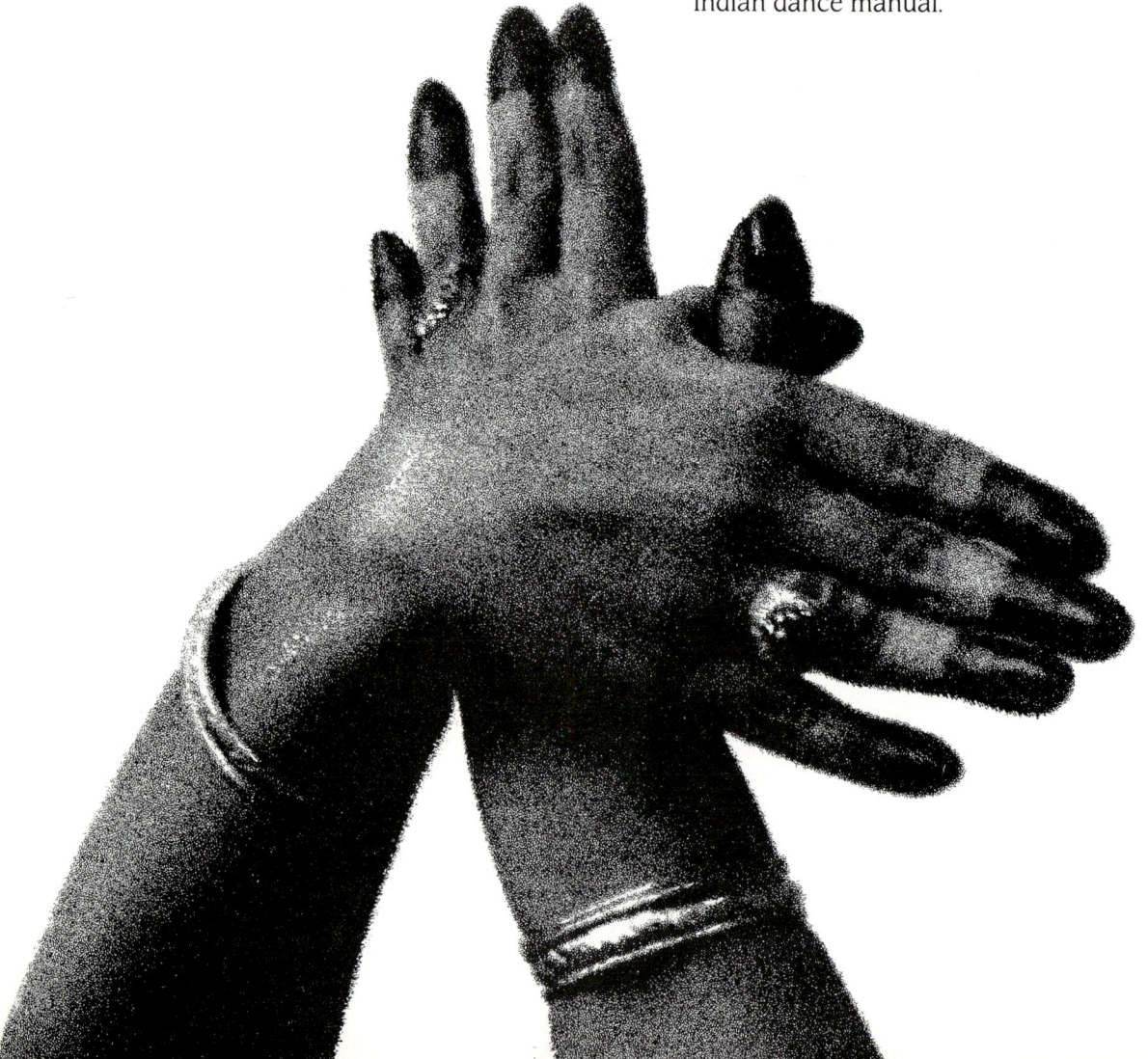

CHAPTER 3

SEDUCTION

Dances of Love

Dance is the language of love. Eager anticipations, bashful adorations, trivial flirtations, foolish promises, absurd escapades, passionate reunions, murderous jealousies, gloomy melancholies, divine bliss, profound despair — all are dialects of this parlance of passion. The contained violence of the flamenco, the voluptuousness of *baladi* dances, the graceful seductiveness of the tarantella, the high-spirited rejoicings of Portuguese dances — all are exaltations of love, whether it be love lost, fulfilled, sacred or impossible.

Tarantella

There are several legends explaining the origin of the tarantella. One is that the dance was invented to heal the bite of the tarantula by sweating out the poison in a frenetic dance. Another charming legend is that the tarantella was created by the Graces. Ulysses, assailed by the sirens' call one day, sealed his ears with wax so that he would not succumb to their charms. Humiliated by his indifference, the sirens went to ask the Graces to teach them seductions irresistible to the King of Ithaca. Out of jealousy or perversity, the Graces amused themselves by demonstrating the tarantella to the poor sirens who could not dance it — and for good reason. Thus, the legend concludes, young women inherited a dance full of grace and gaiety.

Whatever the legends say about the tarantella, it appears that the name is a derivation of Tarento in Italy, the place where, in the time of the ancient Greeks, the dance was likely created.

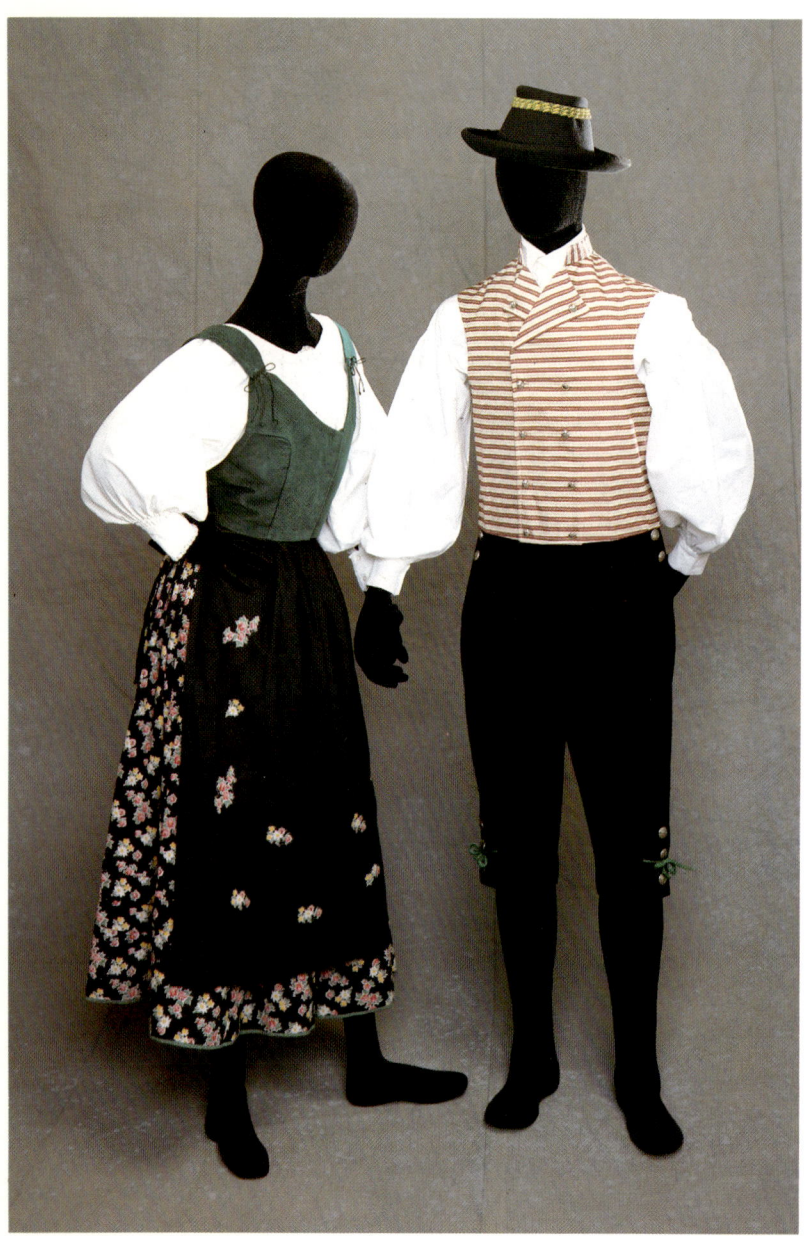

The tarantella is danced throughout southern Italy with significant regional variations. It is a loosely structured dance in which dance steps and figures reflect the mood of the dancer who acts out a scenario clearly evoking games of amorous seduction. It was inevitable that the many southern Italians who emigrated to Canada would bring along the tarantella, an essential element of their cultural heritage.

Tarantella Costumes

These costumes, created in Italy for tarantella dancers, were brought to Canada in the early 1960s. They were worn by the dancers of the All Nations' Rhythmic and Folk Dancers' School in Windsor, Ontario.

Portuguese Dances

Portugal is a country of contrasts. The music of the fado is austere and melancholic but religious fervour, exuberant spirits and soaring passion mark the rich range of other forms of Portuguese cultural expression. Extremely varied rituals of celebration commemorate passage through various stages of life and these rites are deeply rooted in ancestry. Marriage, for example, is the most important celebration of all because it symbolizes the continuing future for the group. Throughout their migrations, the Portuguese have preserved these traditions and, whether in Portugal or in Canada, their culture remains a tapestry in which piety, passion and joy are inextricably interwoven.

Portuguese costumes

The women's costumes of Viana do Castelo in the Minho region are undoubtedly the most colourful in all of Portugal. The brilliance of these costumes is enhanced by the contrast with the men's costumes which are simple and austere.

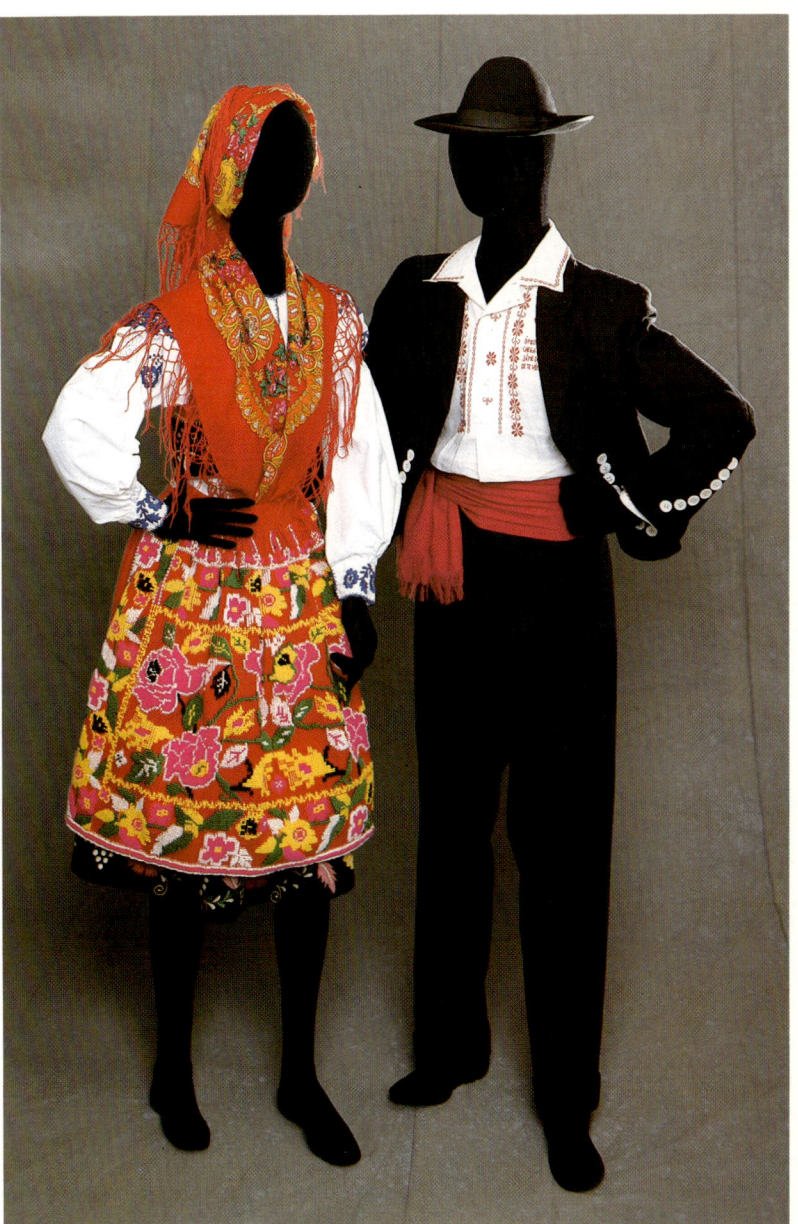

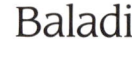

Baladi

To those with only a casual knowledge of Arab dance tradition, the term *baladi* is usually considered synonymous with belly dancing but that art is only one aspect of the complex and subtle choreographic tradition of the Middle East. When the pharaohs reigned, Egypt already had a vast array of ritual dances in honour of Hathor, goddess of love, joy and music. Located on the southern route of Gypsy migrations, Egypt also adopted certain elements of the sacred dances Gypsies brought with them from India. More than anything else, though, Egypt preserved the warm sensuality associated with Arabic culture. With such diverse conditions underlying it, contemporary Egyptian choreography masters the delicate art of seduction in an exemplary manner.

Madame Obadia Dancing the Baladi Accompanied by a Takht Band

Madame Obadia, a Moroccan dancer who specializes in the traditional dances of Cairo, is sparing no effort to re-create in Toronto, her current residence, the most authentic expressions of Egyptian choreographic language. A *takht* band from Toronto accompanies Madame Obadia in the baladi dances. The *takht* is a traditional musical ensemble found in Syria, Lebanon and Egypt. The instruments used are the *ud* lute, the *qanun* zither, the *nay* flute and the *riqq* and *darabukka* drums or *naqqara* kettledrums.

Violut Akili, Darabukka and Naqqara

The lute is the most common musical instrument in the Near and Middle East. Ancestor of the western lute, various forms of the instrument were in widespread use throughout the Islamic world. Designed between 1967 and 1975, this *violut Akili* lute represents a marriage of modern experimental research and the traditional art of lute making.

The Arab *darabukka* drum is used at all celebrations. This highly decorated example is North African.

The *naqqara*, small copper kettledrums played in pairs, are joined by a thong with a lacing of skins surrounding the body of the instrument. They are used in classical and popular Arab music as well as East African music.

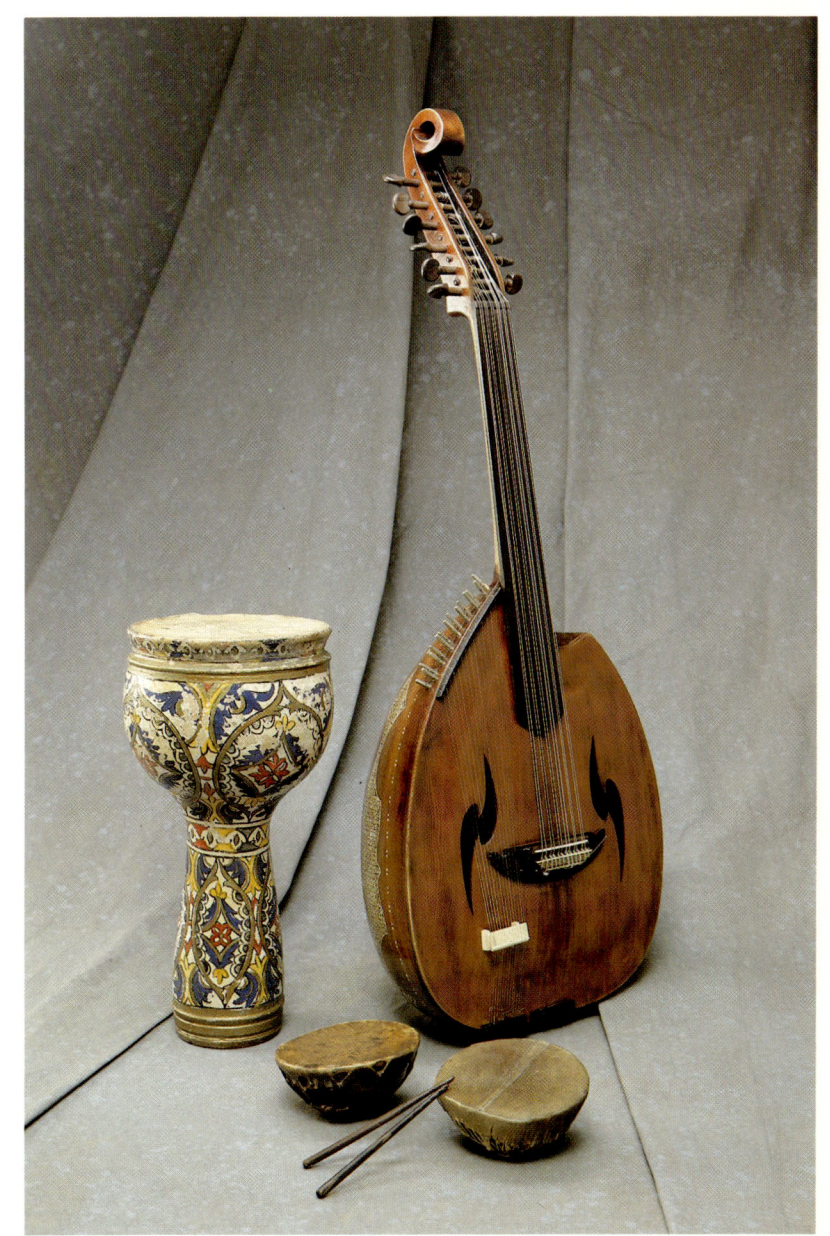

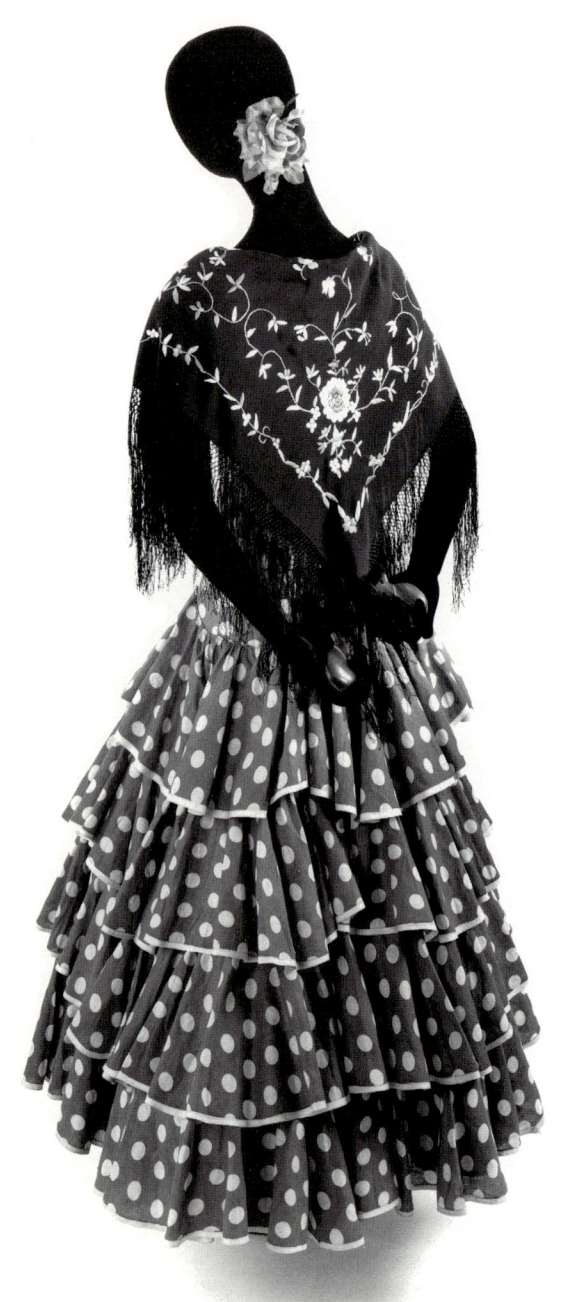

Flamenco

The last Gypsy hordes, expelled from India in 1400 by Tamerlane, had barely begun to settle in Andalusia when, by edict, the King of Castile instituted repression of minority groups in Spain. Gypsies, Jews, Arabs and dissident Christians were forced to take refuge in the mountains and live in hiding for nearly three hundred years. There they sang of their misery and their suffering, their anger and their despair, their hatreds and their loves. Thus, out of passion and distress, was flamenco born.

In 1783, when the Pragmatic Sanction of Charles III permitted these people to come out of hiding, all of Spain was enchanted by the accents and rhythms of flamenco that abruptly burst forth from the mountains. Derived from Gregorian chants, Gypsy dances and Arab and Jewish music, this esoteric art with its enigmatic forms is difficult to export in its original purity. Authentic flamenco is the pure and simple emergence of the soul — naked emotion without modesty or shame. It is a long, sad lament of resignation and a sudden, powerful roar of revolt; a velvety caress of shy tenderness and an intoxication of frenetic passion; the carefree jubilation of freedom and the tragic heartbreak of death. Flamenco is pure passion expressed solely through song, guitar and dance.

Sevillanas Costume

In the cities of Spain, the pressure and fashions of urban lifestyles has transformed the flamenco into the *sevillanas*. The name undoubtedly comes from Seville, the site of the most boisterous annual fair in all of Spain, where city squares and streets echo with contagious rhythms. In Canada, the flamenco is danced primarily in its urban form, the *sevillanas*, usually in Spanish restaurants in the large cities. This dress, with its design of white polka dots on a scarlet background, is a typical *sevillanas* costume.

Flamenco Dancers

A strong bond exists between the flamenco dancer and singer as the dancer transforms into movement the emotions expressed by the singer. Spurred on by the "Oles" of the audience, they encourage each other with glances, snapping fingers (*pito*) and stamping feet (*zapateado*) that express joy or despair, passion or sadness in a crescendo of energy that quickly climbs to thrilling heights of emotional intensity.

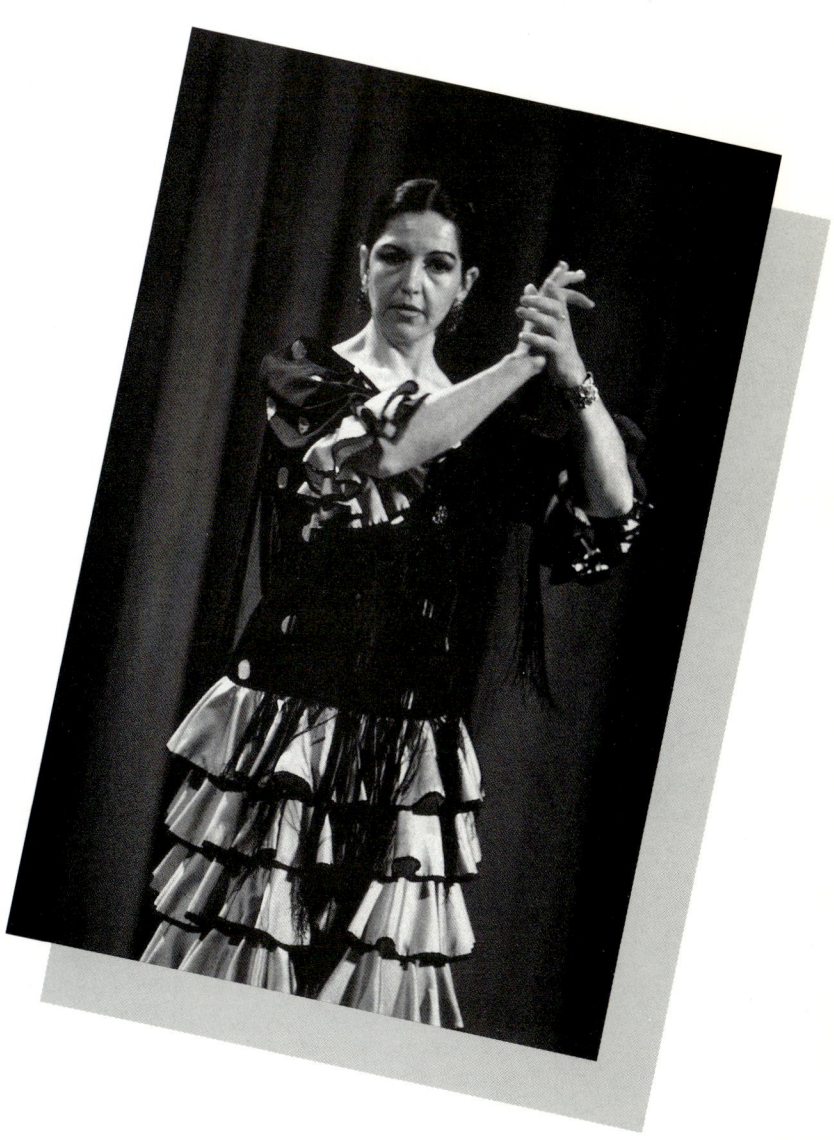

CHAPTER 4

IDENTITY
Dances of Allegiance

Dance as the dynamic image of a group's political and cultural identity is probably the most noticeable social function of dance to emerge in more recent times. For example, the cultural affinities and differences between Baltic and Scandinavian countries are equally expressed in the respective styles of their festive costumes, the shape and decorative designs of their zithers and in the configuration of their dances. Such musical and choreographic traditions as the waltzes and polkas that filled bourgeois salons of Western Europe in the eighteenth century or the *verbunk* danced in Hungary to mock Turkish invaders, stand as incontestable symbols of ethnic and cultural authenticity. In contemporary pluralistic societies such as Canada, traditional music and dances remain the most visible standard of each group's ethnocultural identity.

The People of the Salons

In the late eighteenth century, an extraordinary intermingling of European peoples began. Many travellers left their country's dances as parting gifts and it became fashionable in the great capitals of Western Europe to twirl to the rhythms of foreign dances. This infatuation with novelty threatened the previously unchallenged supremacy of national dances. Minuets and cotillions were gradually replaced by waltzes, polkas, mazurkas and czardas and the movement took hold in North America as well, as seen in the dancing of the varsoviana in Quebec.

Gensliki, Mazanki, and Koziol

The *gensliki* is a small violin carved from a single piece of wood and is found primarily in the Tatras mountains in Poland. It is played alone, or with the *basy* (bass fiddle), to perform folk tunes.

The *mazanki* is a three-stringed violin frequently played with the *koziol* to accompany dances.

Originally from the Tatras region as well, the *koziol*, is a type of bagpipe. The traditional instrument of shepherds, it has a goatskin bag and is generally accompanied with the fiddle or the *mazanki* and, sometimes, the clarinet. The *koziol* is also used at dances.

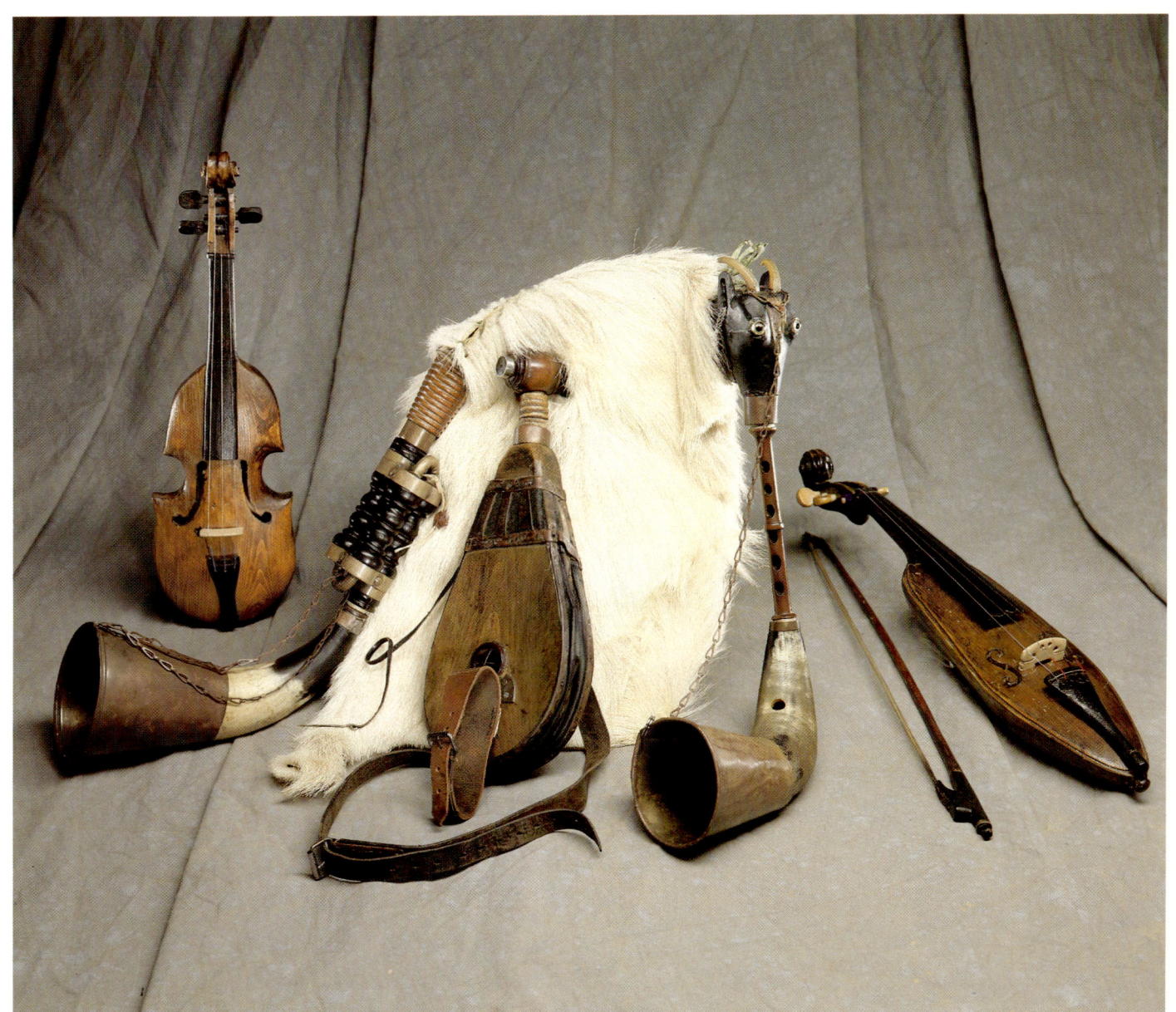

Strings That Bind

Zithers are made from a wide range of materials but all are characterized primarily by strings which are stretched over the length of a soundbox. They are found throughout the world and come in a variety of shapes and sizes. European zithers originally came from the Middle East and those from Northern Europe are often decorated with designs expressing a cosmic vision and recalling the legends and myths of the instrument's creation. The socio-cultural role of the zither is shown most clearly in its musical applications. It can be a folk instrument when used to accompany traditional dances or a classical instrument, as intended by composers such as Liszt, Bartok, Stravinsky or Boulez when they wrote it into their orchestral works.

Zithers made in Canada are inspired by the European model. As well as being used to accompany dancing, the zither in Canada has become the emblem of the vigorous preservation of culture in a new social and political environment.

Langeleik

The Norwegian *langeleik* is a derivation of the Medieval psaltery which came from the Middle East via Spain in the eleventh century. The psaltery underwent constant changes until its final transformation into the harpsichord. The *langeleik* is held on the knees or placed on a table and the strings are plucked with the fingers.

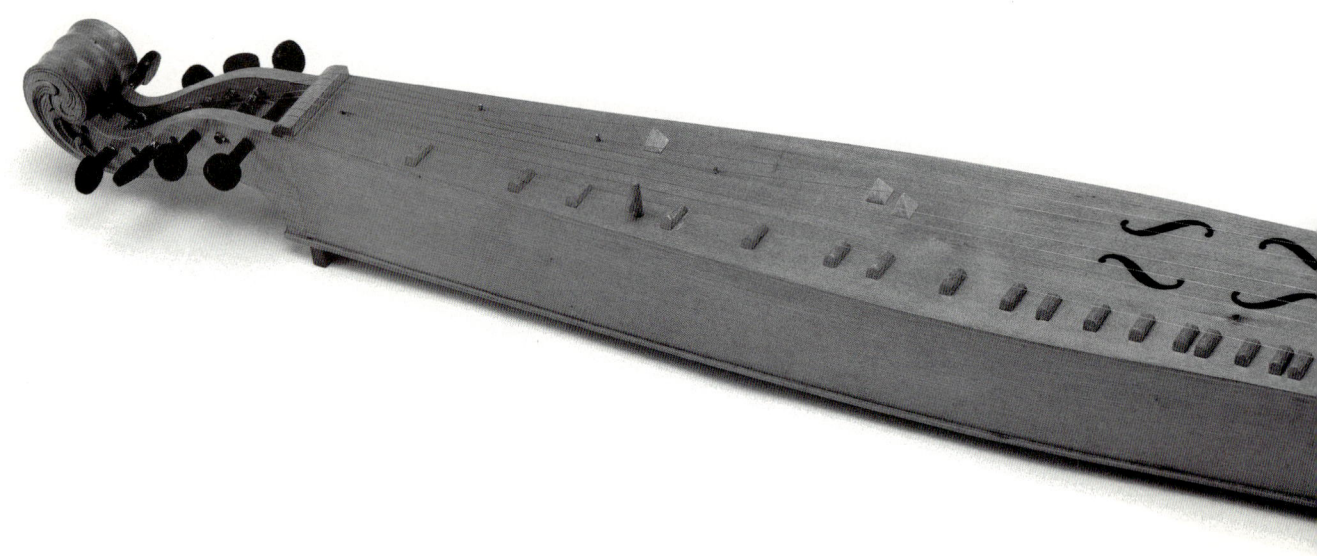

Kokle

The legend surrounding the creation of this Latvian instrument relates to the myth of Orpheus and his ability to command natural forces with his music. In the Latvian legend, the *kokle* possesses the magical power to charm all the animals of the forest and the ornamental designs carved on its sounding board are universal symbols. The circle with a daisy in the middle is a dual symbol of the sun and represents the dynamic force of the heavens and their never-ending rotation. This type of imagery also is found in folk songs and in the movement used in circle dances common to the Baltic countries.

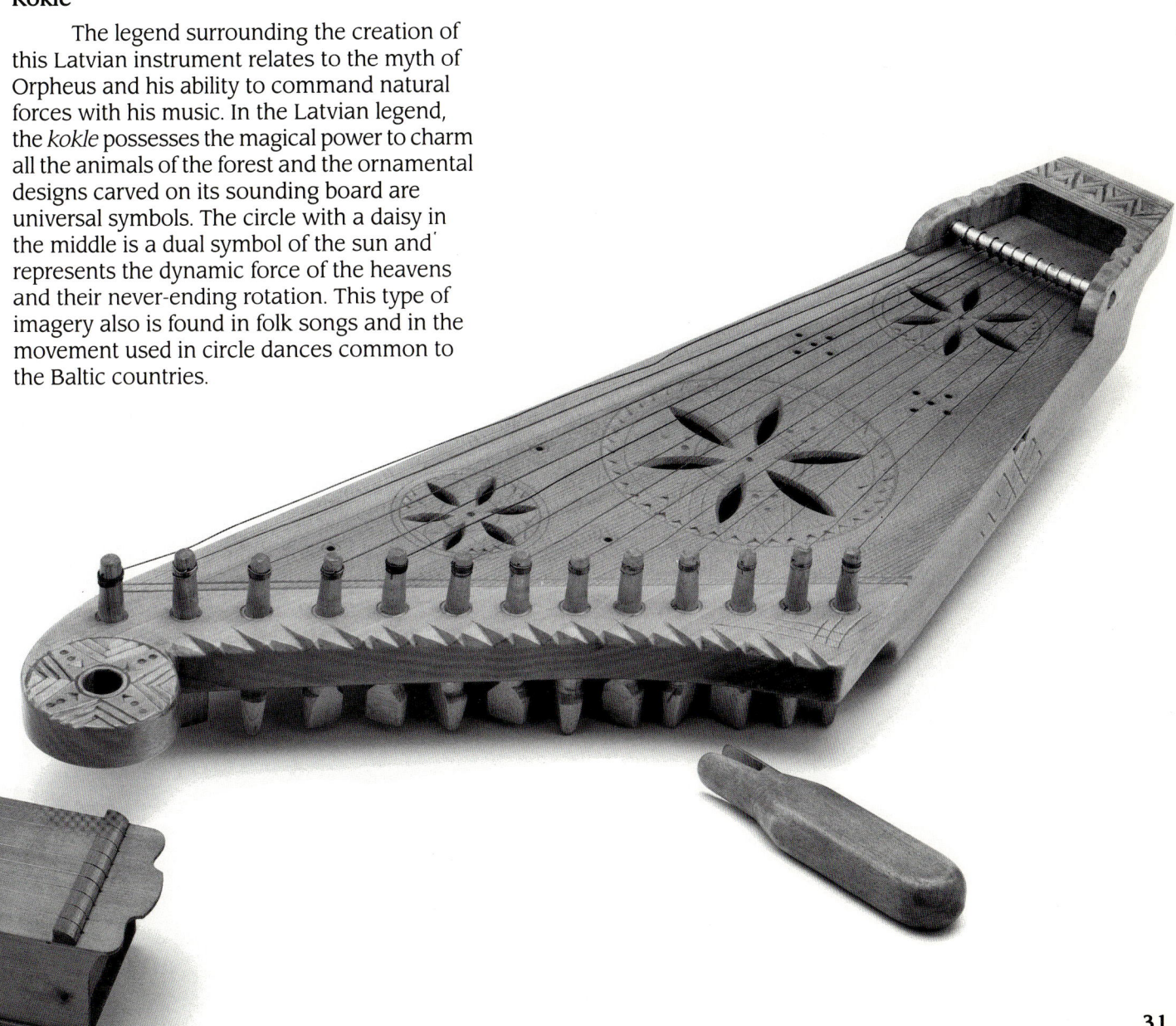

Kankles

Parsidirbau kunklius I made myself a kankles
Ir nuëjau unt kancemu Went down to the inn,
At sisedau unt solelia Sat myself on a bench,
senas bobas karsimau Irritated old women,
Jaunas mergas sokinau But made the young
　　　　　　　　　　　ones dance.

Zilevicius, Juozas. "Kankles mitologijoje, legendose ir tautosakoje pas mus ir musu kaimynus." [Kankles in the mythology, legends, and folklore by us and our neighbors]). *Vairas* 8 (1937): 340-55.

As this traditional Lithuanian song suggests, the *kankles* is used at all social gatherings where there is dancing. It is a faithful companion at all life's milestones — birth, marriage, death. The *kankles* is also used to accompany the *sutartines*, the traditional polyphonic songs of Lithuania. The instrument is placed on the musician's knees, on a table or, to increase its resonance, across an empty barrel.

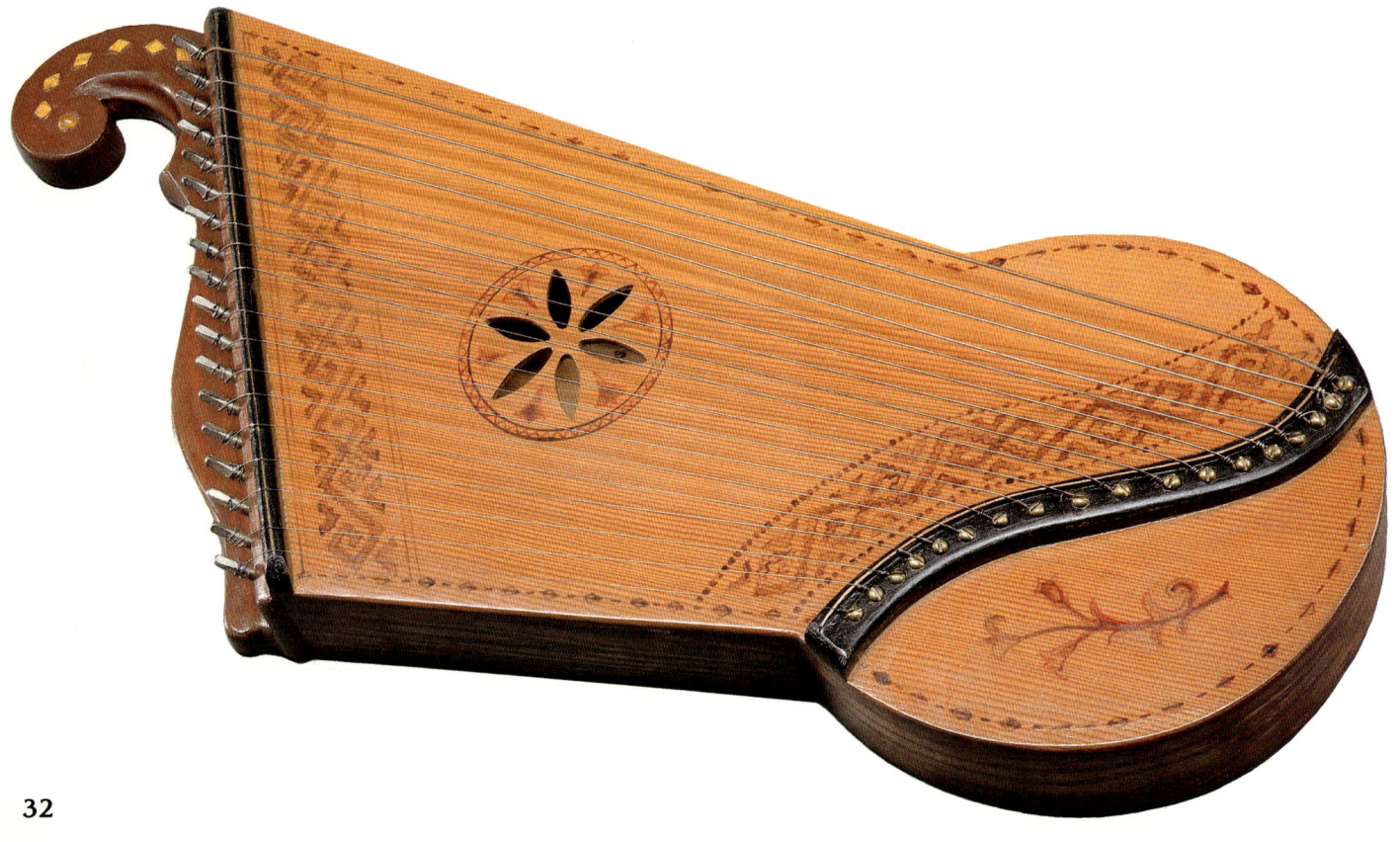

Scandinavian Dance Costumes

The geography of Scandinavian countries creates a distinct and isolated region of Northern Europe. The folklore, traditional dances and national costumes of these countries contain elements distinctive to Scandinavia but parallels also exist in the Baltic countries to the south.

There are similarities in costumes — heavy wool skirts and white blouses and aprons decorated with lace and rich embroidery sewn in geometric patterns and designs of acanthus leaves and snowflakes. Both regions have chain dances and circle dances. They also share common folk festivities. These include the spring festival in celebration of nature's re-awakening after the long winter slumber and the midsummer sun festival in celebration of the night-long light of the northern summer. Songs, music, traditional dances and national costumes are all part of these celebrations.

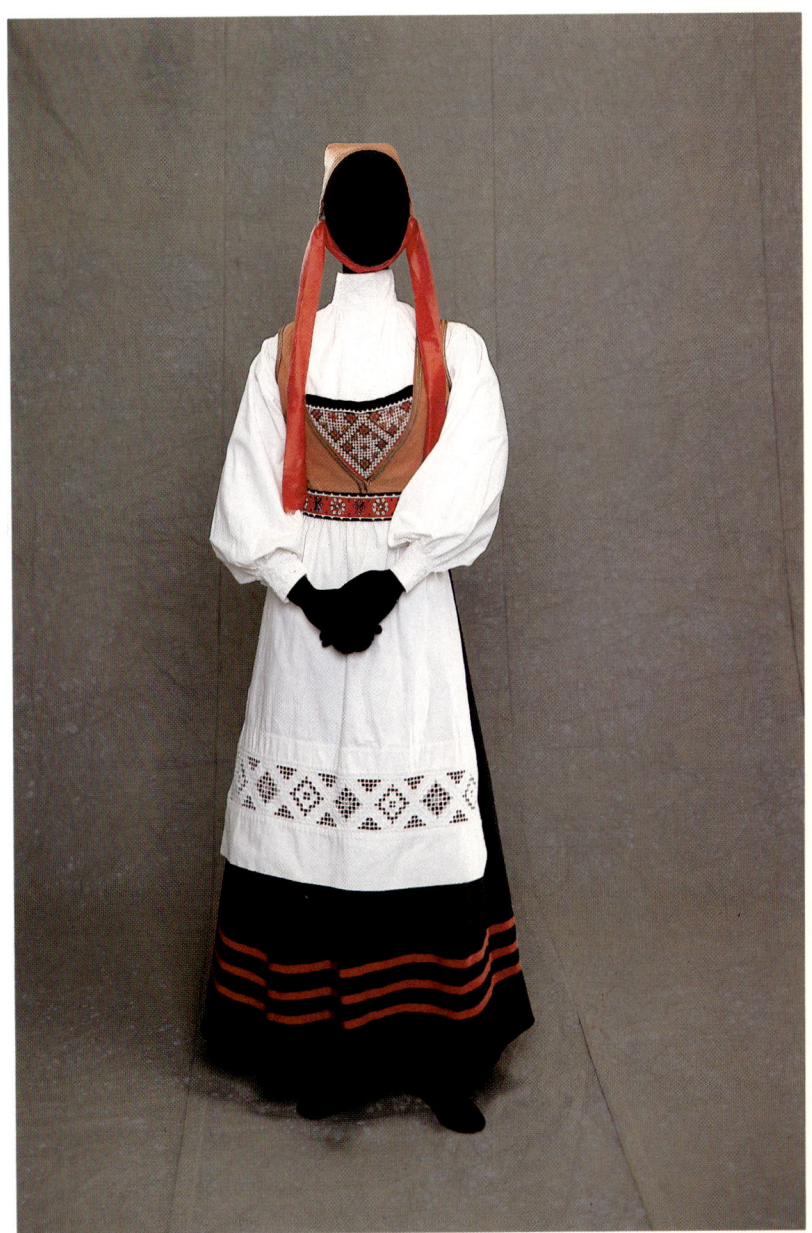

Kantele

The creation of the *kantele* is described in the Finnish epic, *Kalevala*. The legend's hero, Väinämäinen, fashions the instrument using birch for the frame, the teeth of a pike for the pegs and a young maiden's hair for the strings. His skill on the instrument enchants the creatures of the air, the earth and the seas. The *kantele* disappeared from traditional Finnish life after the First World War but, thanks to a folklore revival movement, it reappeared in the sixties and once again enjoys great popularity. The *kantele* is rarely played to accompany dances. It is used primarily to improvise lengthy melodies that accompany the singing of epics.

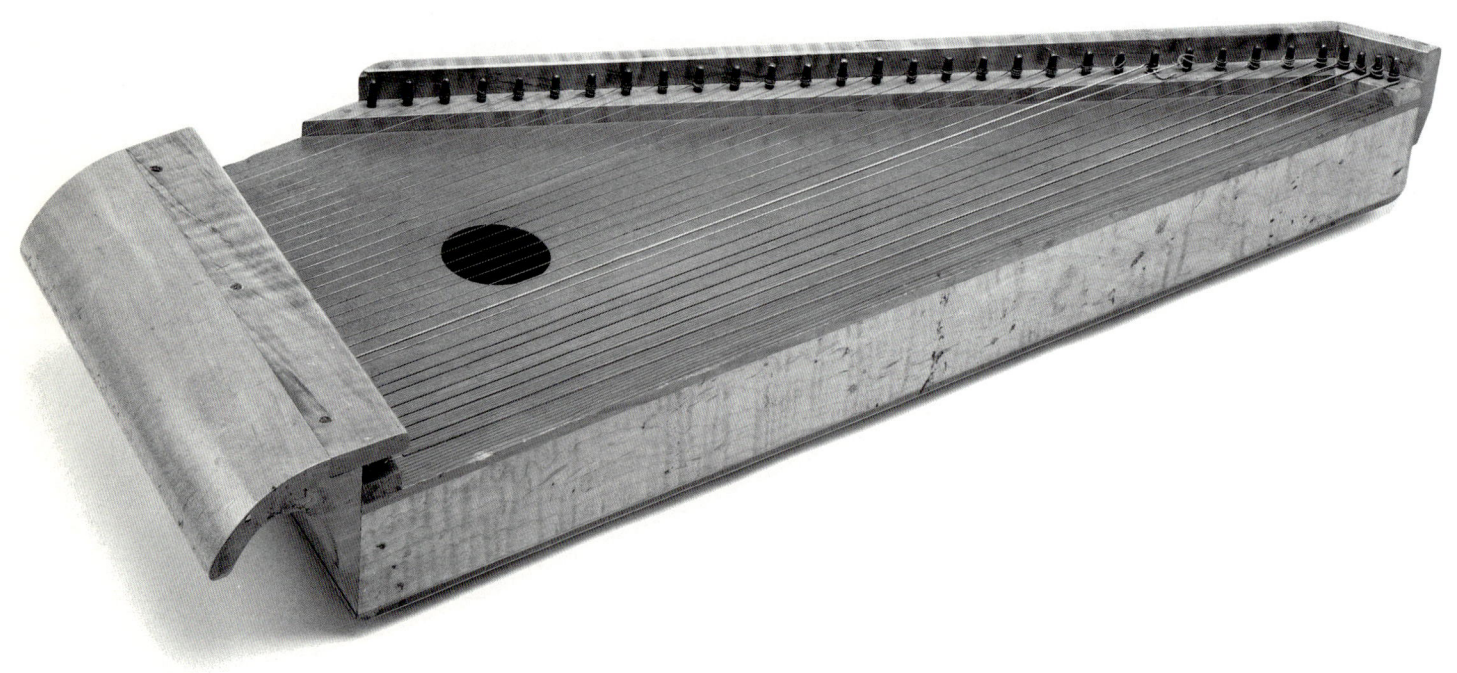

Kannel

A favourite instrument of Estonians, this wing-shaped zither is a variant of the box zither found all around the Baltic Sea. The many strings make it possible to play both melody and accompaniment as the musician plucks melody strings with one hand while strumming with the other to produce chords.

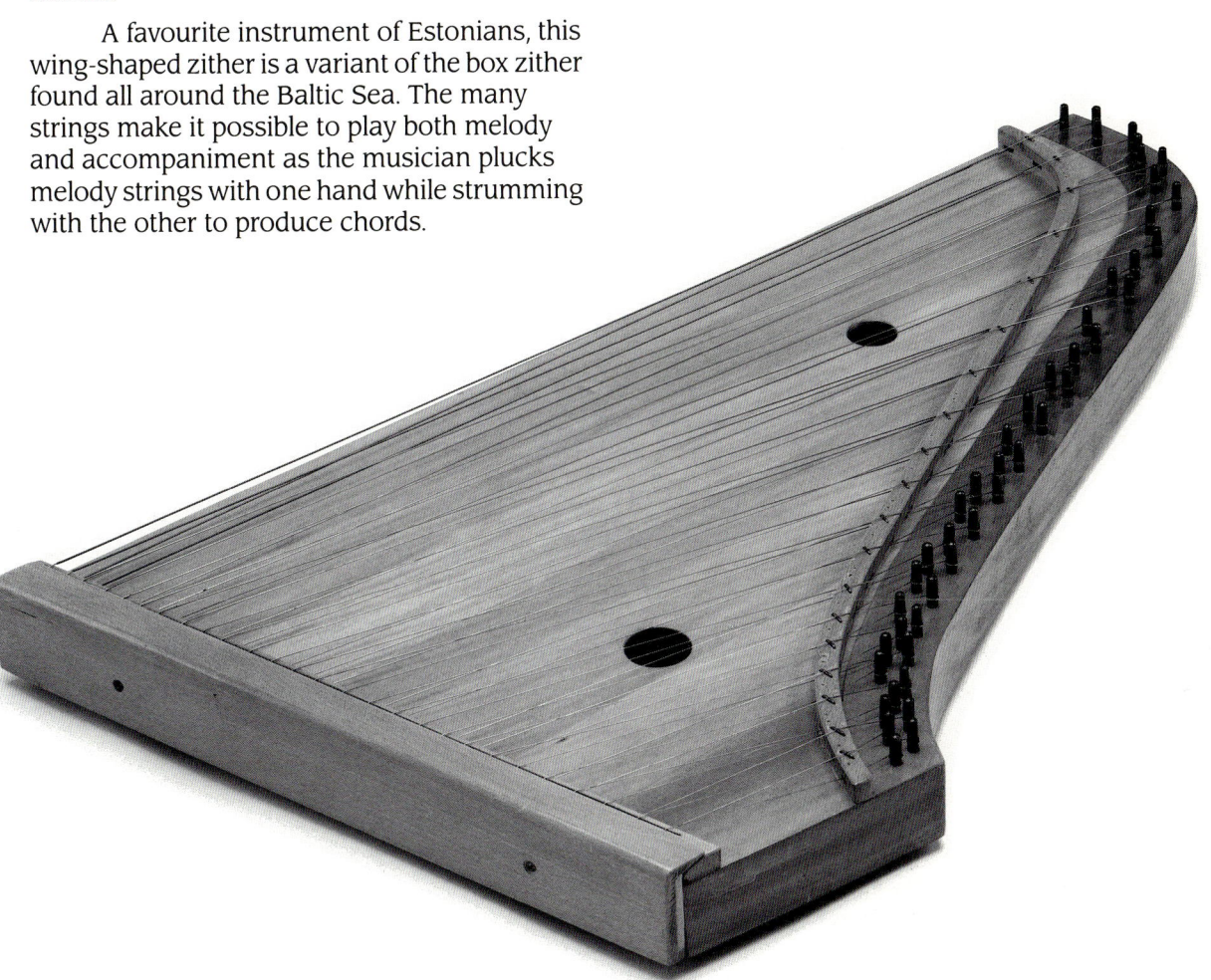

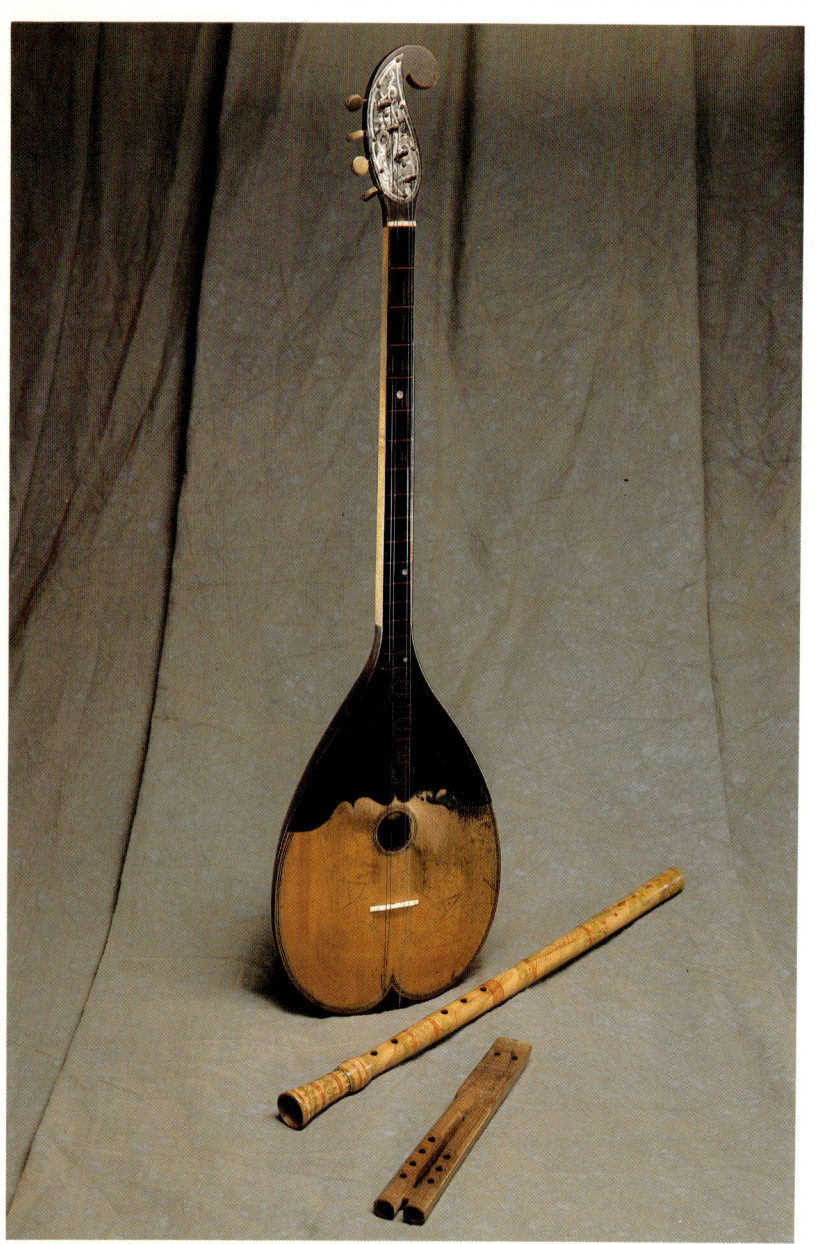

Dances of Resistance

The *hajdu*, *verbunk*, *czardas*, *horos* and *hora* were all originally Carpathian and Balkan peasant dances, probably linked to agricultural fertility cults. Under Turkish occupation, these regions remained isolated from the rest of Europe for many years but the traditional dances were sustained by the political elite as symbols, sometimes even instruments, of resistance to the foreign invader. Over the years, they have become national emblems and remain so, despite migration to Canada. In this country, they bear vivid witness to the ethnocultural identity of the dancers.

Kaval, Dvojnice and Tamburica

The *kaval*, a shepherd's flute, is common in traditional Romanian music and is heard frequently at country fairs and festivals. The player holds it near the lips, blowing across the mouthpiece to produce music of seductive sweetness.

The *dvojnice*, a double flute carved from a single piece of wood, is used in Yugoslavia, especially in the regions of Serbia and Bosnia-Herzegovina where the use of polyphonic vocals is a feature of the local music.

The *tamburica*, a small Yugoslavian lute used as a solo instrument or as part of an instrumental ensemble, accompanies traditional dances and songs. Its characteristic timbre is produced by the playing technique that substitutes a tremolo for sustained notes.

Ukrainian Dance Costume

In the course of their history, the Ukrainians have developed a keen sense of national identity that accompanies them wherever they go and is reflected in their costumes, dances and songs. The women's costumes are especially attractive and distinctive, easily recognized by their geometric designs and beribboned floral headpieces.

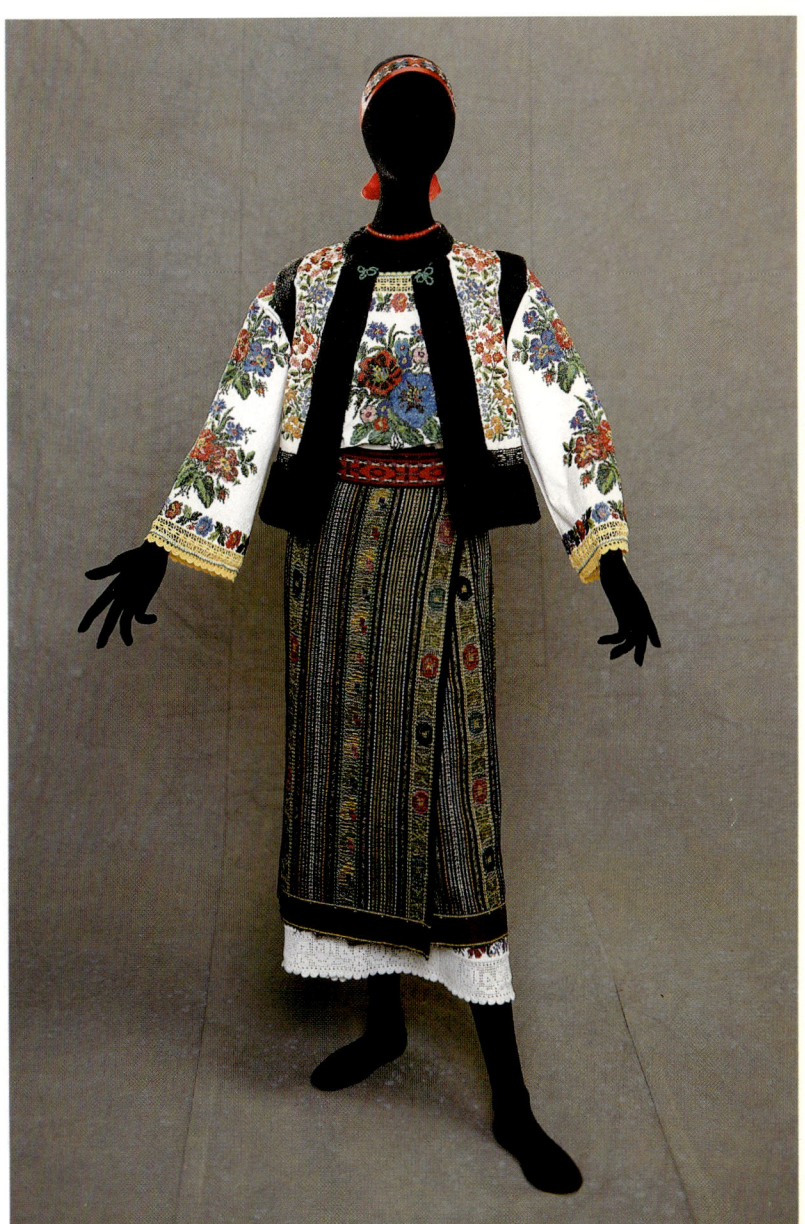

Traditional Hungarian Dance

During community festivals, *legenyes* are danced by young men who stand in front of the musicians and are surrounded by girls waiting to join in the subsequent dances.

The *legenyes* are called "dances of recruitment." Traditionally, these dances were part of the repertoire of herdsmen who were as skilled in the use of weapons as they were in the subtleties of dance. Because of those talents, they became the favourite recruits for the Austrian army in its war against the Turks.

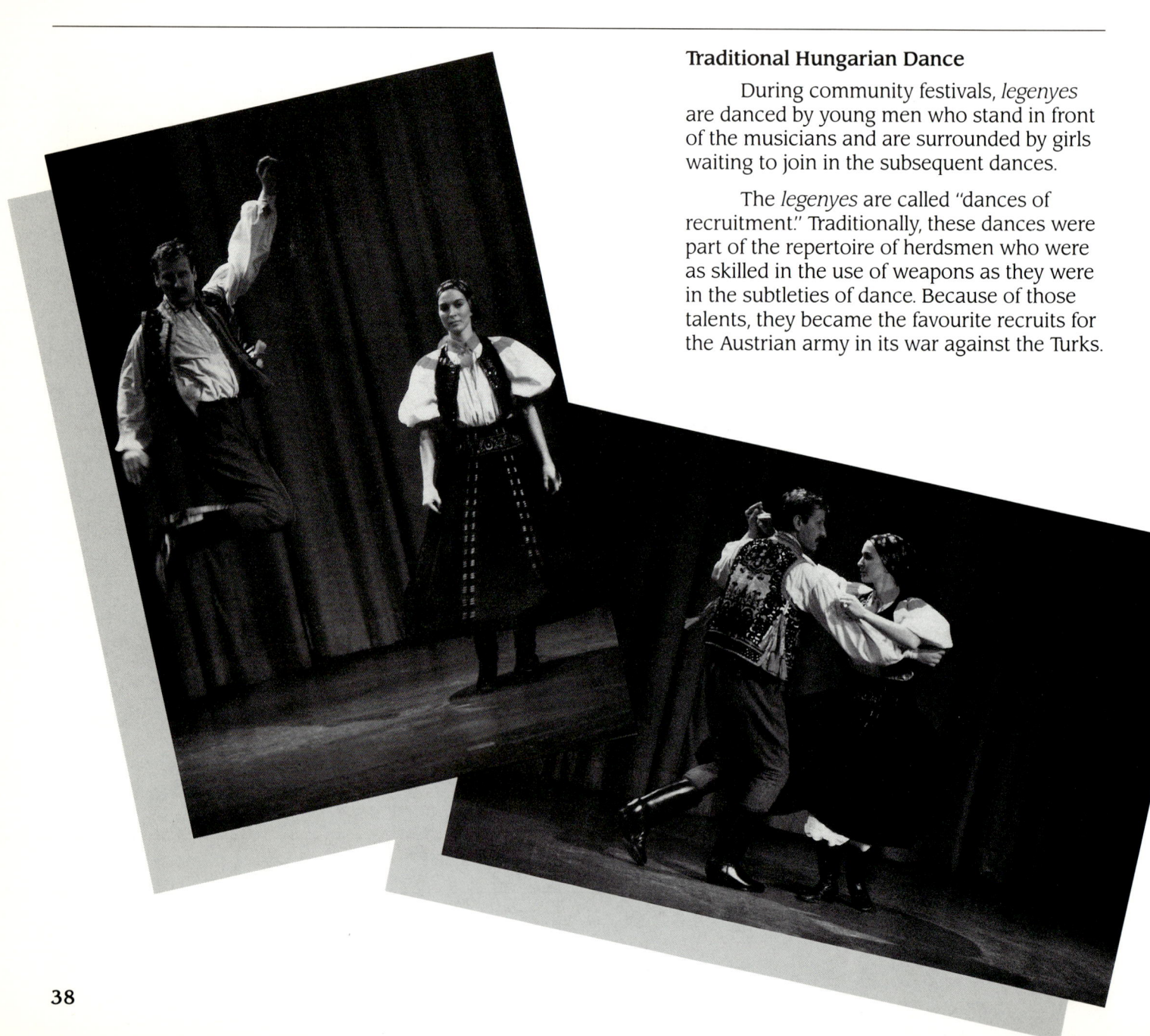

Sopilka

Originally from the eastern and southern Carpathians, the *sopilka* is a very popular end-blown flute in the Ukraine and it is used as a solo instrument or in a group or small orchestra. These particular flutes, brought to Canada in 1948, are engraved with geometric designs of Hutzul origin.

ESCAPISM
Dances of Entertainment

Dance may be a way to communicate with the gods. It may also be the living memory of a community, the language of love and a symbol of national allegiance. It is also pure and simple escapism, however. Dancing allows us to throw off physical and psychological burdens. It diverts us from the cold and gloomy reality of everyday life and introduces us to the imaginary, the fantastic and the carefree. In Canada, dancing is one of the more prominent social pastimes, as shown by the popularity of dance halls and discotheques. From traditional dances handed down from the first settlers to ballroom dancing and the latest contemporary choreographic inventions, there truly is something for every age and taste.

Calypso: The Queen of Caribana

From time immemorial, the carnival has signified a period of abandon in which all excesses are permitted in order to relieve social tensions. In South America and the Caribbean, the carnival has assumed staggering proportions. It is a time of total bedlam, complete licence and monumental extravagance — a time to strut and let loose. Calypso rhythms played by steel bands dominate Carifête in Montréal and Caribana in Toronto, two examples of the Caribbean carnival as imported to Canada. These carnivals take place in summer, not during the winter as tradition dictates, because our winter climate is poorly suited to this type of tropical festivity.

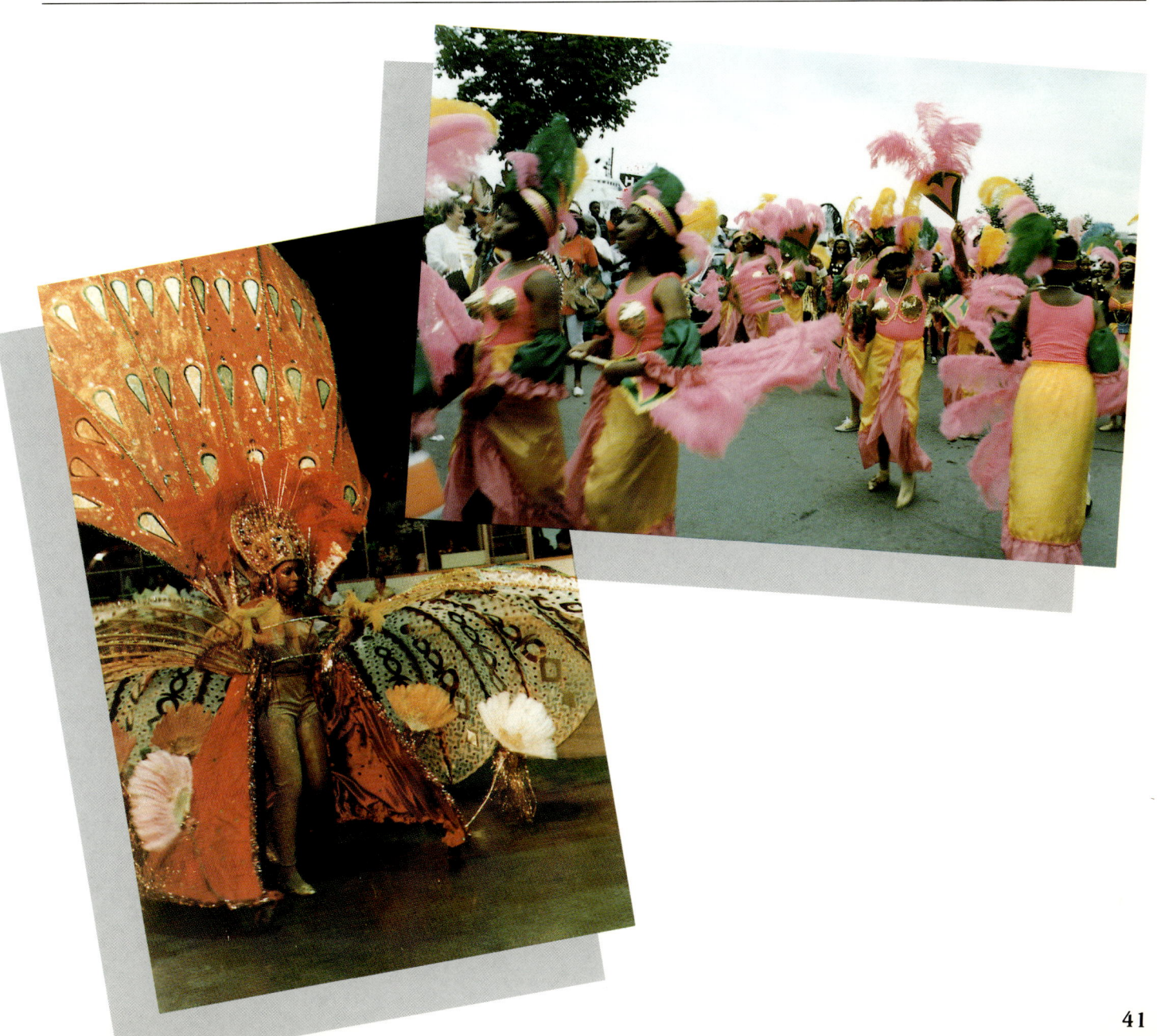

Step Dancing: Donnie Gilchrist

The Ottawa Valley is like a crossroads of traditional dance in Canada. From the meeting of styles as rich as they are varied, a unique style of step dancing has been born. This style is related to the traditional English jig but also displays Amerindian, French Canadian, Scottish and Irish influences, with the American tap dance being a major contributor as well. Donnie Gilchrist made a major contribution to this form of dance and the many dancers trained by him have kept this tradition alive. It continues to this day in all parts of the Ottawa Valley, sustained by the many dance schools that teach step dancing.

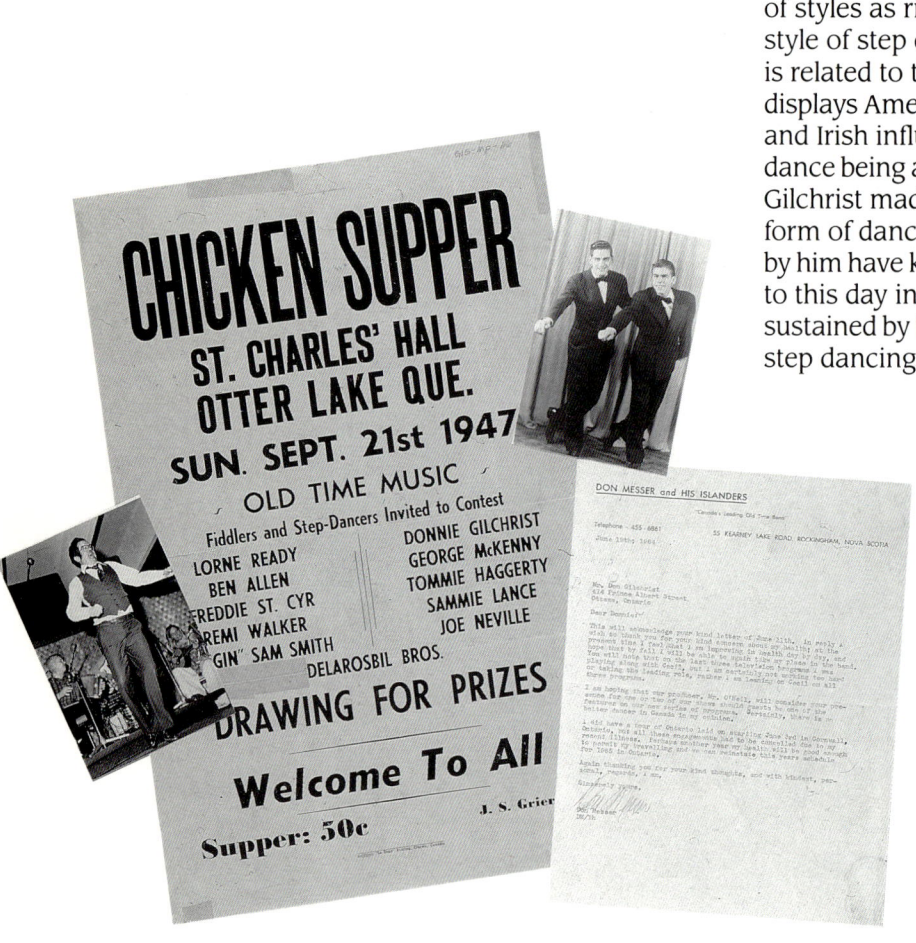

Accordion: Philippe Bruneau

Together with the fiddle, the accordian is a particularly popular instrument to accompany square dances and jigs. Diatonic accordions were first made in Quebec in the early years of this century but before that, they had to be imported from Germany. The instrument was very popular, especially for use in Irish, German and French Canadian music. The latter was enriched by the contributions of such talented musicians as Alfred Montmarquette, Arthur Pigeon and, more recently, Philippe Bruneau.

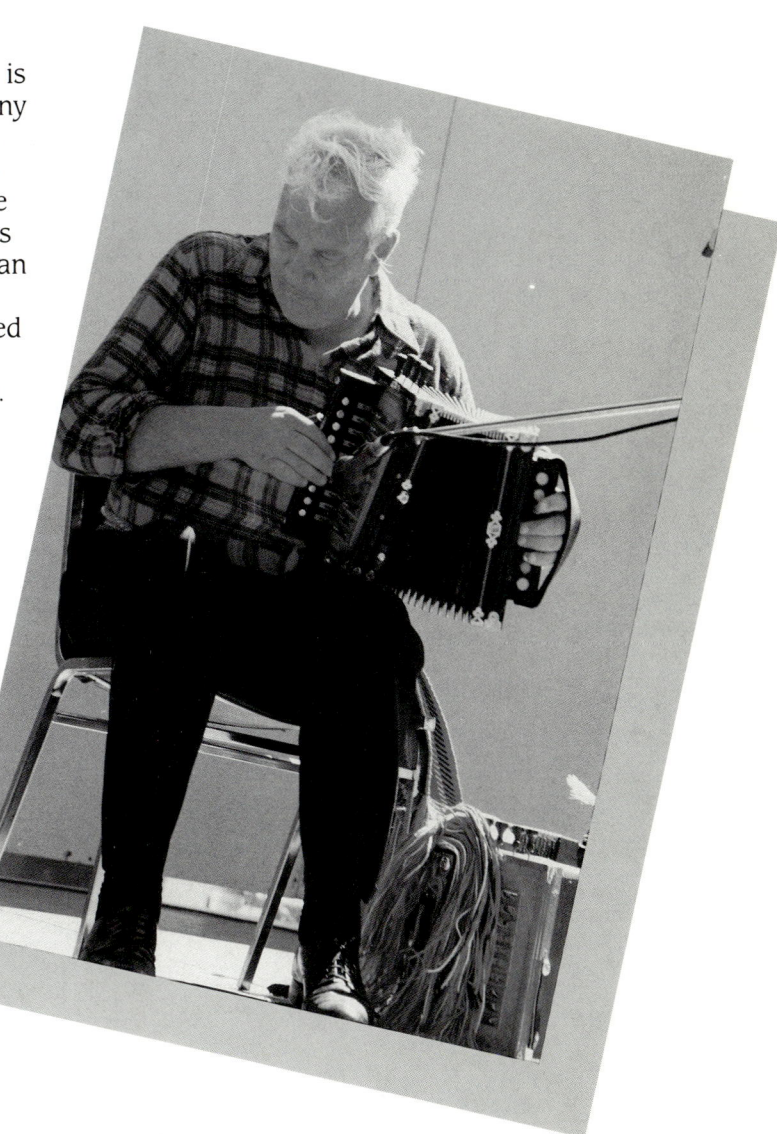

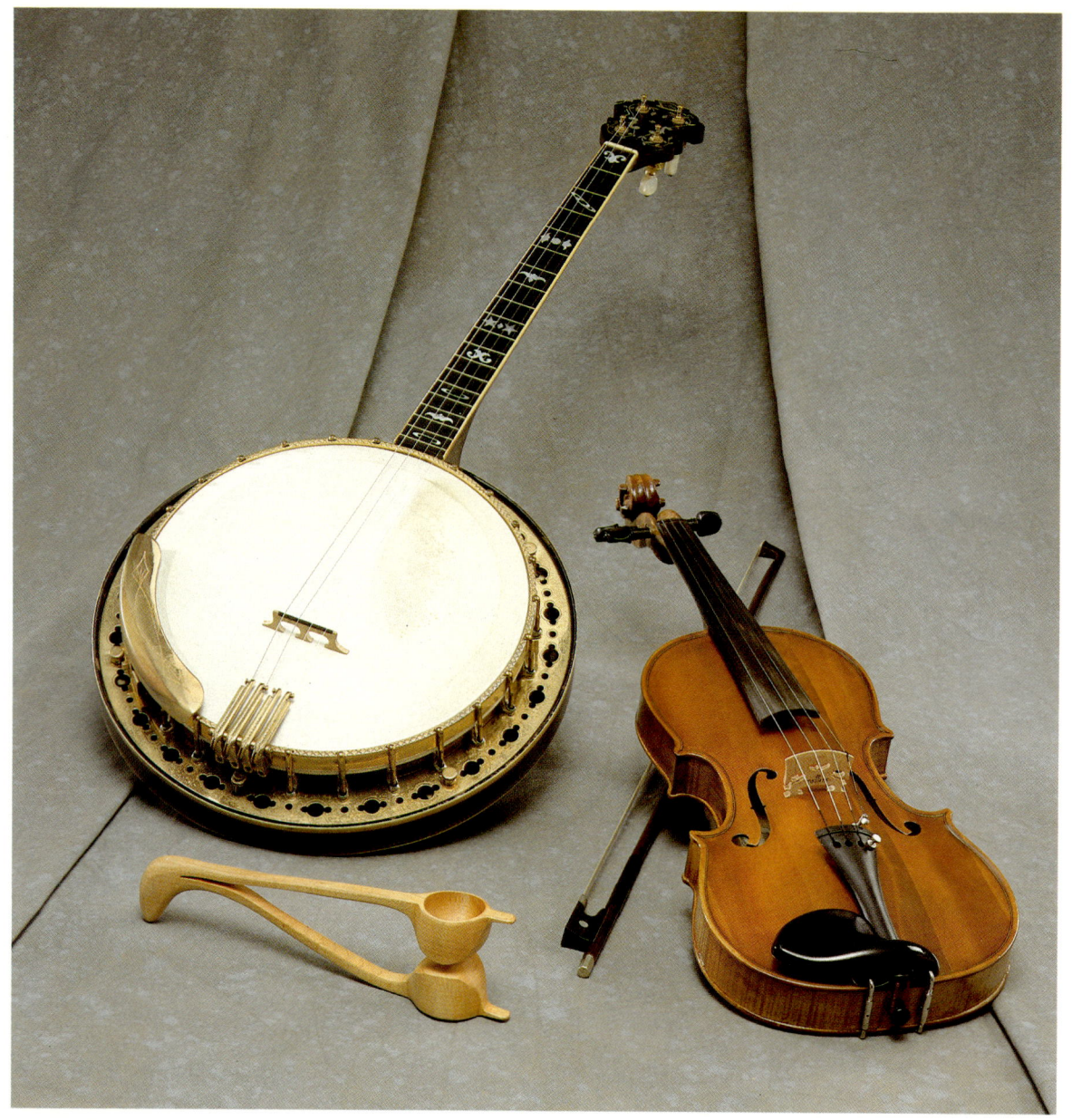

44

Square Dances, Fiddle, Spoons and Banjo

The fiddle is the most popular instrument at square dances in Canada. These traditionally French and English dances, descendants of the ancient chain and circle dances, grew out of the country dances, cotillions and quadrilles brought to Canada by the settlers of the seventeenth and eighteenth centuries. Around 1900, accelerated urbanization made dances for couples especially popular but by 1930, city dwellers had rediscovered the traditional dances which remain popular today throughout the country.

The use of spoons banged together to create rhythmic backup for a melody is universal. However, it was only in the late nineteenth century that this instrument became widely popular in Canada, replacing bones as the rhythmic accompaniment to the fiddle or traditional songs.

The banjo is a modern adaptation of the instrument used by West African slaves in the New World beginning in the seventeenth century. In Martinique, it was associated with the *calinda* dance, later banned by the settlers. Popularized by black minstrels in the United States at the beginning of the twentieth century, it was marketed in its present form in the United States and England. This banjo was built in Canada by a Scots-Canadian around 1933.

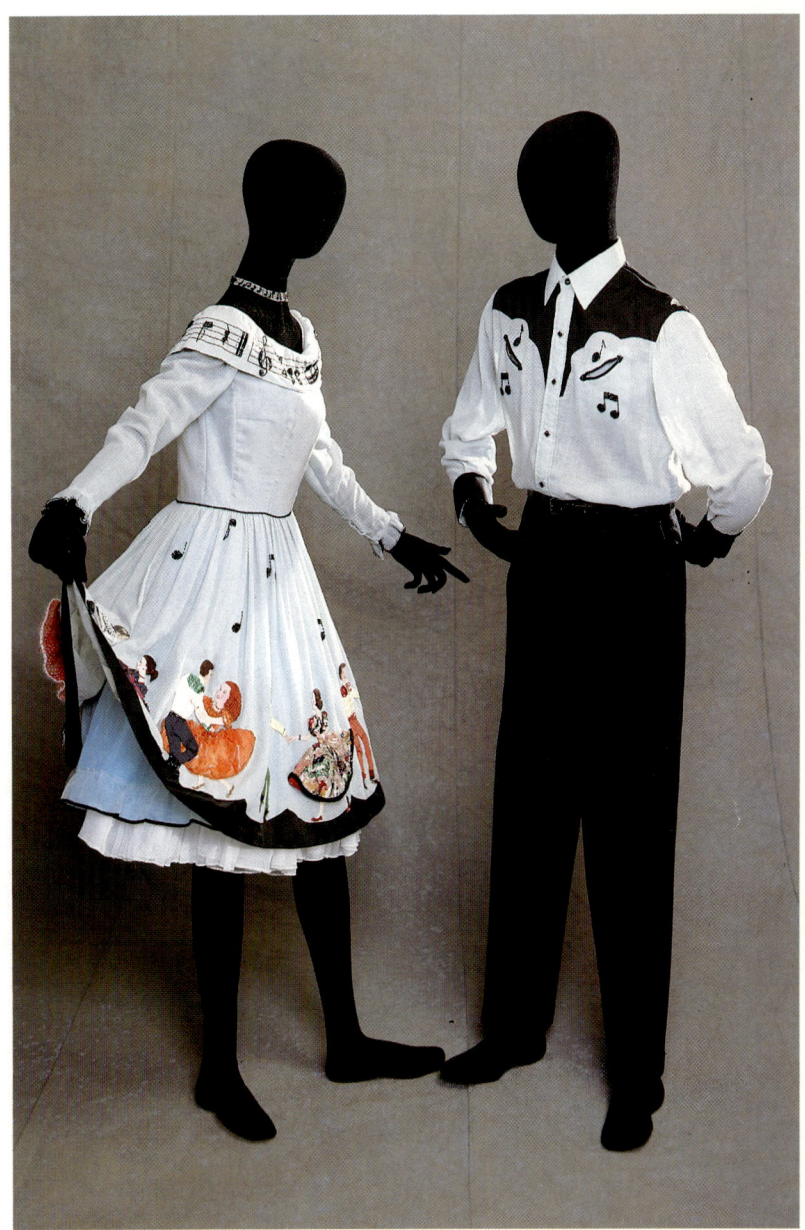

Ballroom Dancing Competitions

The recent tradition of ballroom dancing competitions originated around 1910 when Vernon and Irene Castle opened a dance school in New York and became the darlings of fashionable New York. They set the tone for style with their interpretation of the Argentinian tango they had learned in Paris. The tango became the rage in New York, as it had been in Paris, and was the first Latin American dance to win the public's favour. Others were soon to follow. Vacationers to Cuba in the 1920s brought the rumba back with them and the Brazilian samba was introduced during the 1940 World's Fair in New York. The mambo, merengue and cha-cha followed and are still included in the programs of ballroom dancing competitions. More recently, the advent of such dances as the twist in the 1960s and their subsequent popularity has meant the end of the era when close contact between the dancing couples, a tradition that began with the waltz in the nineteenth century, was what defined formal, ballroom dancing.

Nevertheless, ballroom dancing competitions do remain popular in Canada. The repertoire of ballroom dances is a synthesis of dance styles that, in a hundred years, has gone from everyday locales to ballrooms and back to discotheques. These successive phases reflect the cultural and socioeconomic changes that our society has undergone.

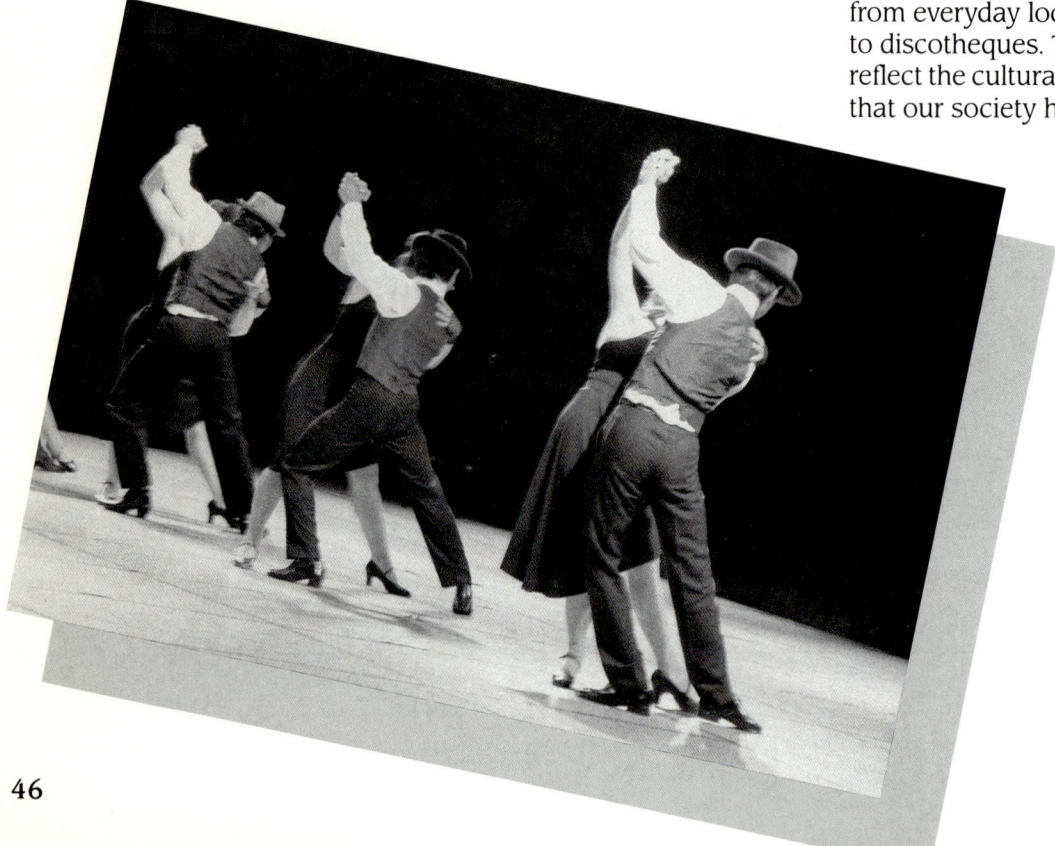

CONCLUSION

PURE PLEASURE

Dance is prayer, thanksgiving, an invitation to love, seduction, an explosion of joy, profound sadness, a dialogue with the gods, an antidote to fear, the recounting of myth or legend, resistance to an invader, communion with the unknown, unbridled playfulness, the magic of acrobatic rhythms and the affirmation of cultural identity. Above all, though, dance is pure pleasure in the fusion of movement with rhythm.

Descriptions of Artifacts and Photos

p. 7 Drum (date unknown)
      Cameroon
      Carved wood
      Height: 160 cm; Diameter: 62 cm
      CCFCS 85-1938

p. 8 Drummer Georges Rodriguez
      and dancer Régine Gilles
      Ottawa, 1987

p. 9 Drum, 1954
      Haiti
      Wood, goatskin, metal
      Height: 99 cm; Diameters: 37 cm and 17 cm
      CCFCS 86-155

p. 10 Mask (date unknown)
      Mmwo tribe (Nigeria)
      Painted wood, fabrics
      Height: 51 cm; Depth: 39 cm; Width: 22 cm
      CCFCS 85-1932

      Kalangu Drum (date unknown)
      Nigeria
      Wood, skin, pebbles
      Height: 37 cm; Diameters: 18 cm and 17.5 cm
      CCFCS 73-1035

p. 11 Mask of Nimba, ca. 1960
      Baga tribe (Guinea)
      Hardwood
      Height: 115 cm; Depth: 39 cm; Width: 30 cm
      CANES B-IV-68

p. 12 Oktoberfest poster, 1986
      K-W Oktoberfest Inc.

p. 13 Hog's Back Morris Dancers
      Ottawa, 1987

p. 15 (left to right)
      Cholera Demon Mask, 1969
      Sri Lanka
      Painted wood
      Height: 76.5 cm; Depth: 15 cm; Width: 59 cm
      CCFCS 81-156

      Garula Mask, 1969
      Sri Lanka
      Painted wood
      Height: 51 cm; Depth: 16 cm; Width: 44 cm
      CCFCS 81-153

p. 16 Udakki Drum, ca. 1960
      Sri Lanka
      Wood, skin
      Height: 24 cm; Diameter: 10.5 cm
      Donated by the Sri Lanka High Commission
      CCFCS 63-14

p. 18 Daisy Sahoo
      Ottawa, 1988

p. 19 (left to right)
      Vina, ca. 1960
      South India Music Emporium, Madras, India
      Wood, steel
      Length: 135 cm; Diameter: 39 cm; Depth: 37 cm
      Donated by the High Commission of India
      CCFCS 62-20

p. 19 Mridanga Drum, ca. 1960
      India
      Wood, skin
      Height: 58 cm; Diameters: 22 cm and 16 cm
      Donated by the High Commission of India
      CCFCS 62-3

p. 20 Mudra: Mythical Garuda Bird
      Vasanthi Srinivasan, Ottawa, 1989

p. 22 Tarantella Costumes, ca. 1960
      Italy
      Women's: cotton
      Men's   : cotton, wool
      CCFCS 89-000

p. 23 Portuguese Costumes (date unknown)
      Minho region of Portugal
      Women's: wool, cotton, sequins,
               CCFCS 77-4
      Men's   : wool, cotton, felt, linen,
               CCFCS 77-2

p. 24 Dahlia Obadia, George Sawa, Ibrahim Eleish
      Toronto, 1987

p. 25 (left to right)
      Darabukka (date unknown)
      North Africa
      Ceramic, calfskin
      Height: 46 cm; Diameters: 23 cm and 14 cm
      CCFCS 73-1045

      Naqqara (date unknown)
      Copper, skin
      Height: 6.5 cm; Diameter: 15 cm;
      Height: 6.5 cm; Diameter: 14.5 cm;
      CCFCS 77-98

      Violut Akili, 1975
      Maher Akili
      Syria and Belgium
      Wood, mother-of-pearl, ivory
      Length: 105 cm; Diameter: 39 cm;
      Depth: 24 cm
      CCFCS 78-399

p. 26 Sevillanas Costume, ca. 1953
      Spain
      Dress and shawl
      Cotton, rayon
      Donated by Mrs. Simonne Voyer
      CCFCS 85-288

p. 27 Boléro: ballet espagnol Montréal Inc.
      Ottawa, 1988

p. 29 (from left to right)
      Mazanki, 1970
      Par Rocholski, Poland
      Wood
      Length: 49 cm; Depth: 4.5 cm; Width: 14 cm
      CCFCS 73-220

      Koziol (date unknown)
      Poland
      Goatskin, copper, walnut
      Height: 100 cm; Width: 44 cm; Length: 76 cm
      CCFCS 67-90